Smart Nutrition Cookbook
& Meal Planner

Chef Marshall O'Brien Group

Smart Nutrition Cookbook & Meal Planner
Chef Marshall O'Brien Group
©2018 Chef Marshall O'Brien Group

First edition

The information in this book not intended to be a substitute for professional medical advice, diagnosis, or treatment. Always seek the advice of your physician or other qualified health provider before beginning a new health regimen.

ISBN 978-0-9966293-8-6

Chef Marshall Press
3440 Belt Line Blvd. Suite 103
St. Louis Park, MN 55416

To order, visit www.ChefMarshallOBrien.com.

Printed in the United States of America

Table of Contents

Introduction   I

The Importance of Meal Planning   3

   Tips for Successful Meal Planning   4

   Batch Cooking Simplifies Meal Preparation   6

   Food Storage Tips   7

   Best Methods for Easy Meals   7

Kitchen Essentials   8

   Pantry Must-Haves   8

   Knives, Pots & Tools   9

Recipes for Quick & Delicious Meals   10

   Breakfast   11

   Lunch   22

   Snacks   33

   Dinner   44

   Slow Cooker & Multicooker Meals   55

   Dressings & Sauces   66

Resources

   Chef Marshall's Meal-Planning Website   73

   The Smart Nutrition Workbook   74

   Meal-Planning Template   75

Conclusion   76

About the Authors   77

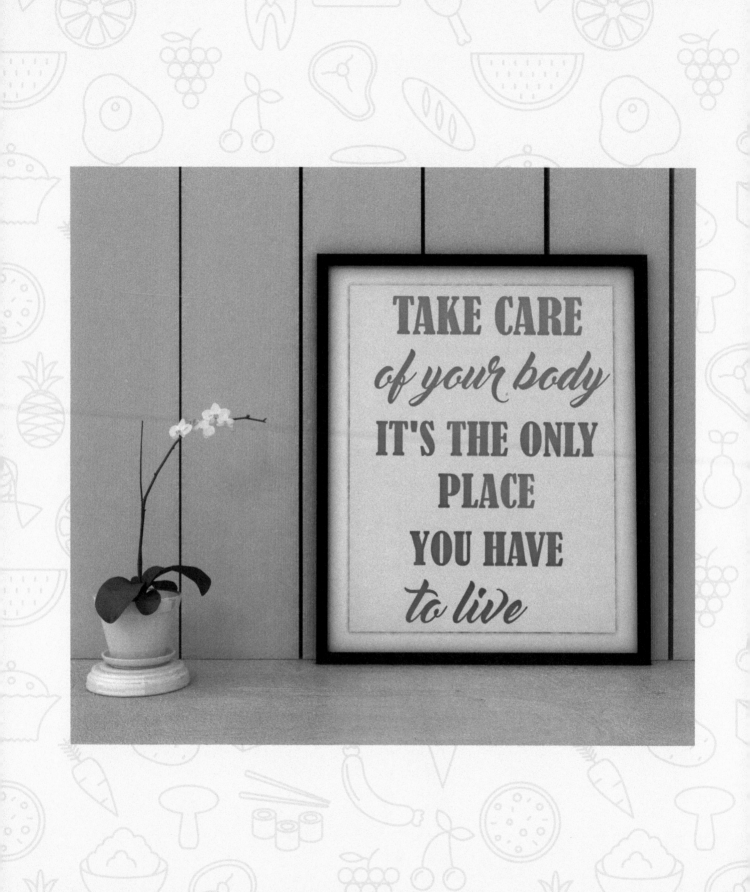

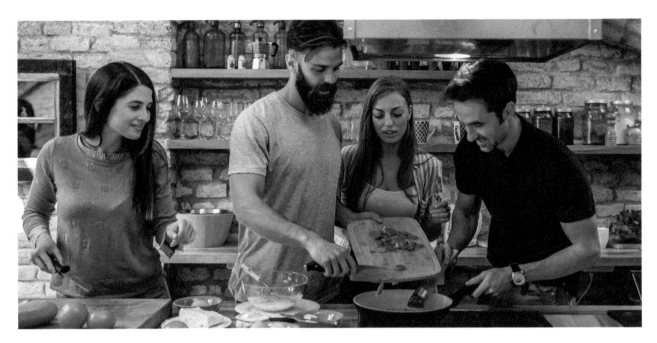

Introduction

Everybody wants to feel better, perform better and live a long, high-quality life.

Think back to the last time you had great energy, sharp mental clarity, low stress and little to no body pain. Wouldn't you like to feel that good again? Wouldn't you like to quit worrying that you might end up with a chronic health condition such as diabetes, arthritis, heart disease or Alzheimer's disease? And wouldn't you like to give your children a healthy start in life? Of course you would and we wrote this book to show you how.

Chef Marshall's Smart Nutrition system provides the pathway, the tools and the guidance for your journey to better health. While every body is different, Smart Nutrition can greatly improve your chances of being healthier and reduce your risk of chronic disease.

The most direct pathway to excellent health is real food, simply cooked and served with love.

Beginning with *The Smart Nutrition Workbook*, we guide you to make better decisions about your health and offer straightforward steps to help you get started.

This book, *The Smart Nutrition Cookbook & Meal Planner,* includes basic recipes that you can make into quick and delicious meals for breakfast, lunch, snacks and dinner.

In addition, this book helps with meal planning, gives cooking and storage tips, and shows how to stock your pantry and equip your kitchen. The tools in this book will help you simplify your life and teach you how to easily prepare the foods you want to include on your journey to a long, high-quality life.

For more recipes and tools, visit our meal-planning website. Learn more about this tremendously helpful resource on page 73.

If you fail to plan, you plan to fail

Benjamin Franklin

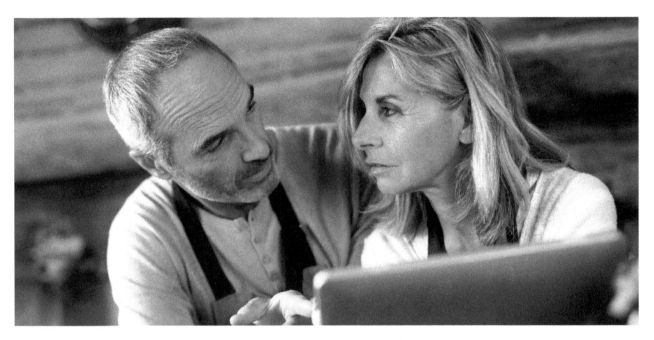

The Importance of Meal Planning

Few things are worse than coming home each night and asking yourself, "What am I going to feed my family tonight?" It puts enormous pressure on you and often leads to your serving foods that are not the best choices, just to complete the task. Now imagine that you have your week's meals and snacks planned so they can be ready in 5-15 minutes when you are under a time crunch. How much stress does that remove from your life? And how much better will you eat?

Smart Nutrition starts with establishing a time each week to plan and begin preparing your entire week's meals, including breakfasts, snacks, lunches and dinners. Many people do this on Sundays, but choose the day that works best for you. Initially this will feel like a major effort, but after a few weeks this exercise will become a normal part of your weekly task list. It will be well worth the time because you will know which meals need to be prepped or cooked in advance due to tight schedules. This advance preparation will allow you to race in after work and "heat and eat" the night's meal when time is short. Here are some more meal planning tips:

- Sleep is just as important as breakfast, so plan simple breakfast foods that can be assembled in five minutes or less. This can be overnight oatmeal, whole grain toast with nut butter, a frozen smoothie or a veggie muffin that was batch-cooked and just needs reheating.
- Package your morning and afternoon snacks in single portion bags so they are ready to grab and go.
- Prepare and package lunches the previous night.
- Prepare dinner or time-consuming components of the meal in advance so you can complete the final preparations and have the meal ready to eat in 30 minutes or less.
- Focus on simple meals or pre-cooked entrees on activity-filled nights. If everyone is not eating at the same time, prepare foods that be kept warm or are easily reheated.

Tips for Successful Meal Planning

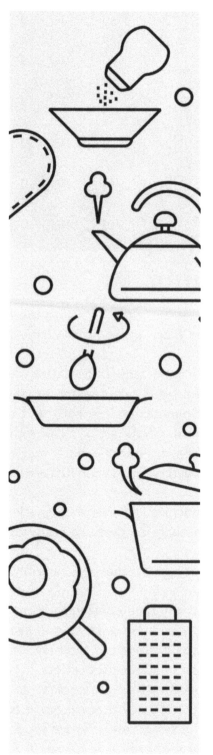

Think Through Your Food Requirements

The best plan is one you will use, so customize your plan by listing each meal and snack you and your family eat during each time frame, as shown below. Meals include breakfast, lunch, snacks and dinner and time frames include weekdays, after school, weekends and special events. Be as specific as possible; add the unique meals and time frames your family deals with, including children's activities, regular activities for you and your spouse and special events, as needed.

For each of these situations that require food, you need to ask: *Will I have time to prepare food OR will I need to make food in advance?*

Breakfast	For my spouse and me during the week For the children during the week For our family on weekends
Lunch	For my spouse and me during the week For the children if they are not eating school lunch For our family on weekends
Snacks	For my spouse and me at work during the week For the children when they come home from school For the children if they are in activities or sports For our family on weekends
Dinner	For our family during the week For the children if they have after school or evening activities For our family on weekends
Special Events	For any member of my family who has regular activities such as a weekly golf game or tennis match or a morning stop at the gym, dance practice or sporting events.

Try our meal-planning template on page 75.

Theme Nights Make Planning Easier

Create an outline that stays consistent from week to week. For example, meatless Mondays, taco Tuesdays, chicken Wednesdays and fish Fridays. Collect recipes that fit these themes and rotate through them. With this method, you avoid repeating the same recipes each week, but don't have to start from scratch every time you put together a new week's plan.

Prep Smart, Cook Fast

Veggies, such as onions, peppers, carrots and other favorites, can be prepped ahead of time for use in roasts and sautés. Pre-cook beans and grains, like rice and quinoa, and freeze them in meal-sized portions. Meats, soups, stews and slow cooker meals all freeze well and are easily thawed for quick meals. Pull items out of the freezer the night before you intend to serve them and thaw thoroughly in the fridge during the day so they are ready to use for dinner.

Keep Fresh Salad Fixings on Hand

Salads are a quick and easy way to get vegetables onto your plate. Rinse, spin and store greens such as spinach, romaine and arugula with a salad spinner so they are ready to go. Top off the greens with cut-up raw vegetables you prepared ahead. These crudités can also be used to accompany lunches or as crunchy midday snacks.

Cook Once, Serve Multiple Ways

Smart meal planners learn to cook in large batches and reinvent the leftovers in delicious ways. For example, here are four meals made with leftover pot roast:

- Portion meat into pita pockets with chopped romaine, a sprinkle of cheddar cheese, chopped tomatoes and a dash of hot sauce.
- Make burritos with avocados and jalapeños.
- Serve with scrambled eggs or in an omelet for breakfast.
- Season with crushed red pepper flakes and serve with a side of warm cornbread.

More Tips

Purchase the right containers so you can store and freeze foods in meal-sized and individual quantities. Portion foods for grab-and-go convenience. Your refrigerator and freezer are your friends.

- Keep on hand breakfast ingredients that can be assembled in two to three minutes or pre-cook foods that only need to be heated.
- Freeze cooked chicken, pork, shrimp or lean hamburgers so you can defrost and heat them as part of your evening meal.
- Set aside time on a weeknight or the weekend to prepare food for the upcoming week. If possible, try to make it a family event.
- Buy some cookbooks with quick and delicious recipes.
- Join a meal-planning website.

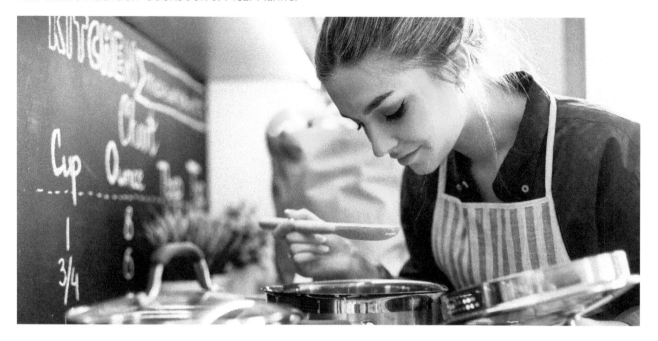

Batch Cooking Simplifies Meal Preparation

Batch cooking is an easy, time-saving way to ensure your family has tasty, nourishing food readily available: cook once, eat several times. For this reason, you should include batch cooking recipes in your menus when you do your weekly meal planning. You will have more food available for the week and you will save time, because you will be cleaning up after preparing fewer meals.

Many of the recipes in this cookbook are excellent for batch cooking. These recipes include tips for make-ahead preparation and storage that will help ensure optimal flavor. You will find these time-saving recipes in every section of the book.

But I Hate Leftovers!

Some people reject the concept of batch cooking, claiming they or their family members do not like to eat "leftovers". However, several meals in this book, such as chicken chili, really do taste better the next day, after the flavors have blended.

Our recipes also suggest ways to prepare in advance some of the more time-consuming ingredients, such as brown rice and ground meat. That way, the final preparation can be done immediately before putting the meal on the table and it's not "leftovers".

Bags of pre-cooked frozen shrimp can be quickly defrosted and sautéed with pre-chopped veggies for a quick stir fry. Chicken breasts, pork chops and hamburgers can be cooked ahead of time (slightly undercooked) and frozen so they are "heat-and-eat" ready.

Fish is Best When Freshly Cooked

Except for foods like tuna salad and frozen shrimp, most fish and shellfish is much tastier and the texture is better when eaten just after it is cooked. We recommend that you prep other components of a fish recipe ahead of time but prepare the fish itself just before it is served. Fish can be refrigerated and enjoyed the next day after very gentle reheating.

Food Storage Tips

Your Freezer is Your Friend

The following recipe ingredients can be purchased and prepared in advance, then stored in your refrigerator or freezer in the portions required for specific recipes.

The following foods freeze well:

Butter - Thaw in the refrigerator before using.

Cooked, seasoned ground meat - Package in recipe-sized portions. Remove from freezer and thaw overnight in refrigerator.

Cooked, seasoned meats - Chicken, turkey, pork and other meats, cut in chunks, as needed. Slightly undercook, since they will be reheated. Remove from freezer and thaw overnight in refrigerator.

Cooked grains - Brown rice, quinoa or other grains, packaged in serving- or meal-sized portions. Remove from freezer and gently heat in a covered pan on stovetop with 1-2 tablespoons of added water.

Cooked whole grain pasta - Package in recipe-sized portions. Slightly undercook before freezing, reheat in a kettle of boiling water for 1-2 minutes, drain and serve immediately.

Chopped herbs - Pack ice cube trays with fresh herbs of your choice, such as parsley, basil, rosemary, oregano, thyme, cilantro, etc. Drizzle olive oil over the herbs and freeze. Remove from ice cube tray and store in resealable baggies. May be added to many one-pot meals while still frozen.

Vegetables - Blends or single varieties. You can wash, chop and freeze fresh produce or buy plain, frozen vegetables on sale.

Stone fruit and berries - Peaches, cherries and other fruits with stones should be rinsed, pitted and chopped. Strawberries, blueberries and raspberries should be rinsed and dried. Lay the fruit in a single layer on a sheet pan and place in the freezer. When frozen, transfer fruit to freezer bags for storage.

Bananas can be peeled and frozen in recipe-sized portions.

Best Cooking Methods for Quick Meals

The cooking methods used in this cookbook are designed to provide quick and easy ways to prepare tasty, nourishing meals. These methods include:

- Stir-frying
- Sautéing
- Roasting or grilling one-pan meals on the stovetop, in the oven or on an outdoor grill
- Slow cooker
- Multicooker (Instant Pot®)

If a recipe suggests using an appliance you do not have, our recipes are designed to be flexible and allow you to use the tools you have on hand. While a specific appliance or tool can make the process easier or quicker, you can still prepare the recipe with basic equipment.

You don't have to invest in a lot of new kitchen equipment to eat well!

Kitchen Essentials

Pantry Must-Haves

Stocking these items in your pantry, spice cupboard, fridge or freezer will mean you can throw together many simple recipes by just buying the protein and specific vegetables needed for the recipe.

While many recipes call for fresh herbs, they can be expensive and may spoil before you can use them. So, unless you have a pot of herbs on your window sill, it's practical to stock your cupboard with dried herbs so you aren't scrambling to add flavor to your food.

Pantry/Refrigerator

Apple cider vinegar
Balsamic vinegar
Black beans, low-sodium, canned
Brown rice
Butter (store in freezer)
Diced tomatoes, canned
Eggs
Extra virgin olive oil
Ketchup
Kidney beans, low-sodium, canned
Lemon juice
Lime juice
Mayonnaise
Garlic, minced, in olive oil
Mustard, Dijon
Mustard, yellow
Nut butter
Olive oil
Onions, yellow or white
Quinoa
Rolled oats
Sriracha or Tabasco sauce
Sweet potatoes
Tuna fish, in water or olive oil
Broth, vegetable or chicken, low-sodium, no added ingredients
Whole grain pasta

Herbs and Spices

Basil, dried
Black pepper
Cardamom, ground
Chili powder
Cinnamon, ground
Cumin
Dill, dried
Garlic, granulated
Ginger, ground
Onion powder
Paprika
Parsley, dried
Rosemary, dried
Salt, kosher or sea
Thyme, dried leaf
Turmeric
Vanilla extract

Extras

Almond extract
Bay leaves
Ginger, fresh (store in freezer)
Fresh herbs, as needed
Frozen berries (for smoothies)
Lemons, fresh
Limes, fresh
Tomato salsa

Knives, Pots & Tools

Experienced home cooks usually have cupboards and drawers stuffed with specialty pans and gadgets that can intimidate the novice cook. It is not necessary to spend a fortune on all this equipment when you are starting out. Instead, buy some basic equipment and, as you gain experience and figure out which cooking methods you enjoy and suit your lifestyle, gradually add to your inventory.

Even if your family is small, keep in mind that larger pans will be helpful for batch cooking.

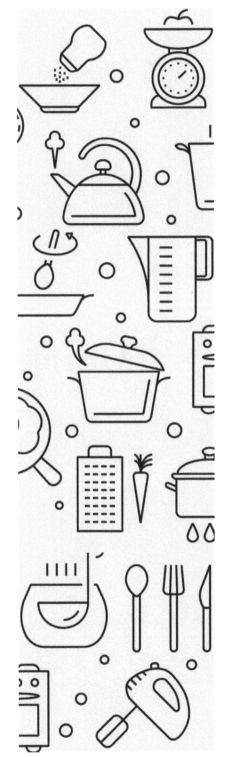

Utensils

Can opener
Grater
Colander
Cooling rack
Cutting board for produce and
    cooked food
Cutting board for raw meats, fish
Freezer containers,
    individual and meal-sized
Kitchen scissors
Ladle, 6-ounce
Measuring cups
Measuring spoons
Mixing spoons
Mixing bowls, large and small,
    metal or glass
Rubber spatula, heat-resistant
Serving fork (large)
Slotted spoon
Strainer/sieve
Food thermometer, oven-safe
Tongs
Vegetable peeler
Wire whisk

Knives

8-inch chef's knife
Boning knife
Knife sharpener
Paring or utility knife
Serrated knife

Pots & Pans

1-quart sauce pan
5- or 6-quart stock pot
9- or 10-inch skillet
12-inch skillet
1 or 2 sheet pans with 1-inch sides

Small Appliances

Blender (stand or stick)
Multicooker
Slow cooker
Toaster

"Nice to have" items

2-quart sauce pan
Food processor
Food scale
Steamer
Fish spatula (long and wide)
Spice grinder
Honing steel for knives
Mixer (stand or hand)
Salad spinner
Microplane® grater or zester

Recipes

for

Quick & Delicious Meals

Breakfast

Breakfast is the most important meal of the day. When you wake up, you have gone 10-12 hours without food, your metabolism has slowed and your fuel tank (energy supply) is low. Breakfast is the meal that gets your day off to a good start.

Like all meals, breakfast should include lean protein, slow carbohydrates and healthy fats.

Since we believe getting enough sleep is critical, we have designed these meals to minimize the morning prep time required. They can be made in minutes or made ahead in batches so all you need to do is heat-and-eat at home or grab them from the refrigerator on your way out the door.

Overnight Berry Oatmeal

Makes 2 servings

Make-Ahead Tip
The texture of this oatmeal is best when eaten within 1-2 days.

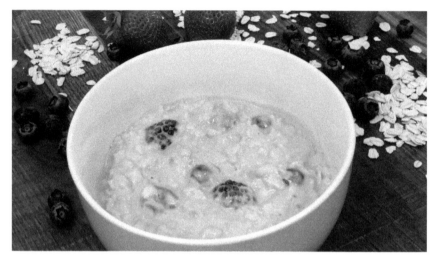

Ingredients
1 cup old-fashioned rolled oats
1 cup plain Greek yogurt, regular or low-fat
1 cup unsweetened almond milk
¼ teaspoon almond, or vanilla extract
4 teaspoons pure maple syrup or honey
1 cup frozen mixed berries, thawed

Directions
1. Thoroughly combine oats, yogurt, almond or vanilla extract, and maple syrup or honey.
2. Refrigerate overnight.
3. In the morning, stir in berries and enjoy.

Nutrition Facts
Overnight Berry Oatmeal

Amount Per Serving

Calories 355	Calories from Fat 54
	% Daily Value*
Total Fat 6g	9%
Saturated Fat 1g	5%
Cholesterol 5mg	2%
Sodium 233mg	10%
Potassium 170mg	5%
Total Carbohydrates 56g	19%
Dietary Fiber 11g	**44%**
Sugars 15g	
Protein 14g	28%
Vitamin A	12%
Vitamin C	2%
Calcium	64%
Iron	23%

* Percent Daily Values are based on a 2000 calorie diet.

Cardamom Ginger Quinoa Bowl

Makes 4 servings

Make-Ahead Tip
Keeps well in refrigerator for 4-5 days.

Grab-and-Go Breakfast

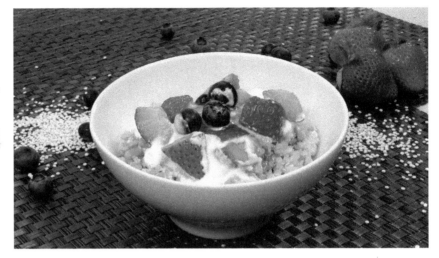

Ingredients

1 cup dry quinoa
2 cups water
½ teaspoon ground ginger
½ teaspoon ground cardamom
⅛ teaspoon kosher salt
1½ cups plain Greek yogurt, regular or low-fat
4 tablespoons honey
1 cup blueberries, blackberries, raspberries or strawberries
½ cup unsalted, raw almonds, chopped

Directions

1. Combine quinoa, water, ginger, cardamom and salt in a sauce pan. Bring to a boil, reduce heat to low, and cover.
2. Cook quinoa mixture for 15 minutes. Remove from heat, let rest for 5 minutes and fluff with a fork. Quinoa can be made ahead of time and chilled.
3. To serve, evenly distribute quinoa into 4 bowls. Top with yogurt, honey, berries and almonds.

Nutrition Facts

Cardamom-Ginger Quinoa Bowl

Amount Per Serving

Calories 346	Calories from Fat 99

	% Daily Value*
Total Fat 11g	17%
Saturated Fat 1g	5%
Polyunsaturated Fat 1g	
Monounsaturated Fat 1g	
Cholesterol 37mg	12%
Sodium 90mg	4%
Potassium 349mg	10%
Total Carbohydrates 43g	14%
Dietary Fiber 5g	20%
Sugars 9g	
Protein 18g	36%
Vitamin A	1%
Vitamin C	7%
Calcium	18%
Iron	27%

* Percent Daily Values are based on a 2000 calorie diet.

Sweet Potato Black Bean Burrito

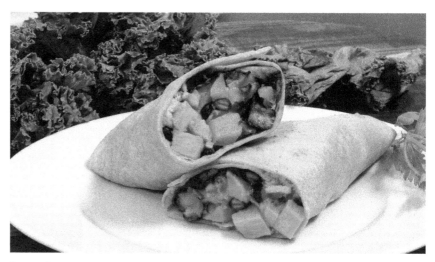

Makes 6 servings

Make-Ahead Tip
To make ahead, omit avocado and salsa garnish, individually wrap burritos and place in the freezer. The night before you want to eat them, remove from the freezer and place in refrigerator to thaw. The next morning, warm in the microwave for about 1 minute.

For grab-and-go, package salsa and diced avocado (drizzled with lime or lemon juice to prevent browning) in small serving cups.

Option: Roast sweet potatoes in advance.

Ingredients
4 whole wheat tortillas
2 tablespoons olive oil
6 cups sweet potatoes, diced
3 tablespoons butter
8 large eggs
1 teaspoon cumin
½ teaspoon oregano
1 teaspoon minced garlic
2 15-ounce cans black beans, rinsed and drained
⅔ cup shredded mozzarella cheese
½ cup low-sodium salsa
2 avocados, diced, optional
Salsa for garnish, optional

Directions
1. Preheat oven to 450 degrees. Line a baking sheet with foil or parchment paper.
2. Toss diced sweet potatoes in olive oil and roast in oven for 15-20 minutes.
3. In a medium bowl, whisk eggs, cumin, oregano and garlic.
4. Heat a skillet on medium heat. Melt butter and cook eggs, stirring occasionally. When eggs are halfway done, add black beans, cooked sweet potatoes, cheese and salsa.
5. If serving immediately, spoon the warmed filling down the center of each tortilla, top with avocado and salsa; fold in the edges and roll up tortillas.

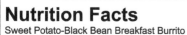

Nutrition Facts
Sweet Potato-Black Bean Breakfast Burrito

Amount Per Serving

Calories 384	Calories from Fat 135
	% Daily Value*
Total Fat 15g	**23%**
Saturated Fat 6g	**30%**
Polyunsaturated Fat 1g	
Monounsaturated Fat 6g	
Cholesterol 228mg	**76%**
Sodium 389mg	**16%**
Potassium 421mg	**12%**
Total Carbohydrates 44g	**15%**
Dietary Fiber 11g	**44%**
Sugars 6g	
Protein 17g	**34%**
Vitamin A	292%
Vitamin C	6%
Calcium	13%
Iron	13%

* Percent Daily Values are based on a 2000 calorie diet.

Turkey Sweet Potato Hash

Makes 4 servings

Make-Ahead Tip
Cool before packaging in individual portions. Freezes well.

Grab-and-Go Breakfast

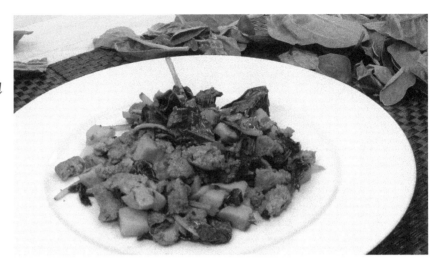

Ingredients

2 tablespoons olive oil, divided
1 pound sweet potatoes, peeled and diced
1 pound lean ground turkey
½ cup yellow onion, diced
5 ounces fresh spinach, chopped
½ teaspoon kosher salt
1 tablespoon fresh thyme, minced

Directions

1. Heat 1 tablespoon olive oil in a large skillet on medium-high heat and add sweet potatoes.
2. Cook over medium heat until golden brown and soft, about 7-8 minutes. Stir every 1-2 minutes. Remove potatoes and set aside.
3. Add 1 tablespoon olive oil to the skillet; add turkey and cook through while breaking into pieces.
4. Add onions and cook until softened, about 4-6 minutes, stirring occasionally.
5. Add spinach, salt and thyme; cook until spinach is slightly wilted.
6. Add cooked sweet potatoes and heat through.
7. Garnish hash with a dollop of Lemon Cumin Yogurt Sauce. (page 70).

Nutrition Facts
Turkey Sweet Potato Hash

Amount Per Serving

Calories 302	Calories from Fat 135

	% Daily Value*
Total Fat 15g	23%
Saturated Fat 3g	15%
Polyunsaturated Fat 1g	
Monounsaturated Fat 5g	
Cholesterol 65mg	22%
Sodium 289mg	12%
Potassium 482mg	14%
Total Carbohydrates 19g	6%
Dietary Fiber 3g	12%
Sugars 4g	
Protein 24g	48%
Vitamin A	279%
Vitamin C	23%
Calcium	7%
Iron	18%

* Percent Daily Values are based on a 2000 calorie diet.

Chicken, Broccoli & Potato Strata

Makes 6 servings

Make-Ahead Tip
Pre-portion this dish in individual servings for an easy, well-balanced breakfast.

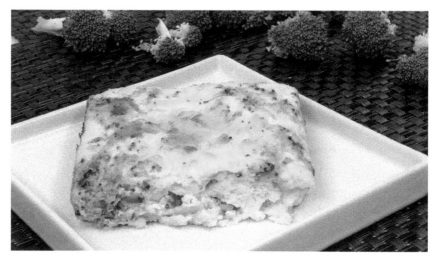

Ingredients
2 tablespoons butter

¾ pound leftover roasted vegetables like broccoli, cauliflower, asparagus, potatoes, chopped

½ pound leftover cooked chicken, chopped

¼ teaspoon salt

¼ teaspoon black pepper

12 eggs

½ cup shredded Parmesan cheese, optional

Directions
1. Preheat oven to 350 degrees.
2. In a large bowl, whisk the eggs until light and fluffy.
3. Grease a 9x13-inch glass dish. Layer with vegetables, chicken and half of the Parmesan cheese, if using.
4. Pour whisked eggs over vegetables and chicken, then sprinkle with the remaining Parmesan cheese.
5. Bake until golden brown and cooked through, about 40-45 minutes.
6. Cool slightly before serving.

Nutrition Facts
Chicken, Broccoli and Potato Strata

Amount Per Serving

Calories 279	Calories from Fat 153

	% Daily Value*
Total Fat 17g	26%
Saturated Fat 6g	30%
Polyunsaturated Fat 2g	
Monounsaturated Fat 6g	
Cholesterol 467mg	156%
Sodium 418mg	17%
Potassium 329mg	9%
Total Carbohydrates 6g	2%
Dietary Fiber 2g	8%
Sugars 2g	
Protein 25g	50%
Vitamin A	73%
Vitamin C	18%
Calcium	9%
Iron	14%

* Percent Daily Values are based on a 2000 calorie diet.

Green Eggs & Ham Muffins

Makes 8 servings, 3 muffins each

Make-Ahead Tip
Cool and package individual servings for grab-and-go breakfasts. Muffins will keep in the fridge for several days and may be frozen.

Grab-and-Go Breakfast

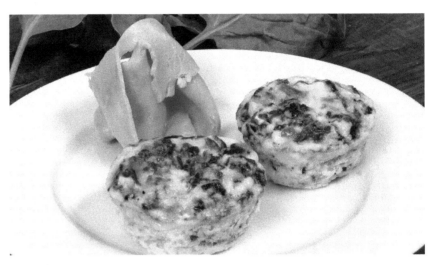

Ingredients
3 tablespoons unsalted butter
½ cup onion, minced
16 ounces all natural, nitrate-free ham, diced
8 cups spinach, chopped (5-ounce package)
16 large eggs
¼ teaspoon black pepper

Directions
1. Preheat oven to 350 degrees. Use a non-stick 12-cup muffin pan. Grease with butter or olive oil. *
2. In a large sauté pan, heat butter over medium heat. Add onions and ham and cook until onions are soft and ham is browned, about 5-6 minutes.
3. Stir in spinach, turn off heat and cool slightly. Spinach should be partially wilted.
4. Whisk eggs and pepper; add to onion, ham and spinach mixture.
5. Ladle mixture into muffin cups, filling to ¼ inch below top. Bake 20-22 minutes, until eggs are set.

Nutrition Facts	
Green Eggs and Ham Muffins	
Amount Per Serving	
Calories 205	Calories from Fat 135
	% Daily Value*
Total Fat 15g	23%
Saturated Fat 6g	30%
Polyunsaturated Fat 1g	
Monounsaturated Fat 5g	
Cholesterol 316mg	105%
Sodium 166mg	7%
Potassium 291mg	8%
Total Carbohydrates 2g	1%
Dietary Fiber 1g	4%
Sugars 1g	
Protein 16g	32%
Vitamin A	46%
Vitamin C	10%
Calcium	6%
Iron	11%
* Percent Daily Values are based on a 2000 calorie diet.	

*We don't recommend using paper liners for this recipe, as they tend to stick to the egg mixture.

Wild Rice, Mushroom & Egg Muffins

Makes 6 servings, 2 per serving

Make-Ahead Tip
Freezing may soften texture slightly.

Grab-and-Go Meal

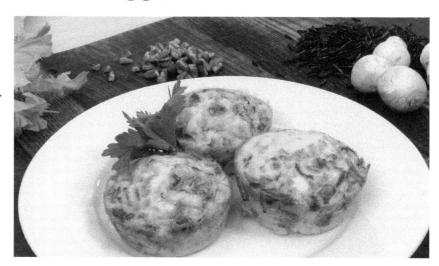

Ingredients

½ cup dry wild rice
2 tablespoons olive oil
8 ounces crimini or button mushrooms, diced
1 tablespoon garlic, minced
1 cup yellow onions, minced
1 cup celery, minced
6 eggs, beaten
6 ounces Gruyere or Swiss cheese, shredded
¼ cup pecans, toasted and chopped, or other nuts of choice
¼ cup parsley, chopped
⅛ teaspoon salt

Directions

1. Preheat oven to 350 degrees. Grease a 12-cup muffin pan.
2. Cook wild rice per package directions; cool to room temperature.
3. Heat olive oil in a sauce pan on medium heat; add mushrooms garlic, onions and celery and sauté until softened, 5-7 minutes. Cool to room temperature.
4. In a large bowl, combine wild rice, mushrooms, cooked vegetable mixture, eggs, cheese, pecans and parsley; mix well.
5. Scoop the mixture into the muffin cups and bake until golden brown, about 20-25 minutes. Cool for 10 minutes before serving.

Nutrition Facts

Wild Rice, Mushroom and Egg Muffins

Amount Per Serving

Calories 326	Calories from Fat 189

	% Daily Value*
Total Fat 21g	32%
Saturated Fat 8g	40%
Polyunsaturated Fat 3g	
Monounsaturated Fat 9g	
Cholesterol 238mg	79%
Sodium 115mg	5%
Potassium 387mg	11%
Total Carbohydrates 17g	6%
Dietary Fiber 2g	8%
Sugars 3g	
Protein 18g	36%

Vitamin A	16%
Vitamin C	10%
Calcium	33%
Iron	10%

* Percent Daily Values are based on a 2000 calorie diet.

Zucchini Carrot Muffins

Makes 12 muffins

Grab-and-Go Breakfast

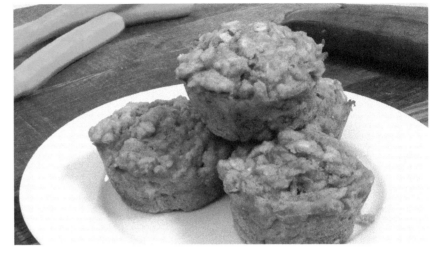

Ingredients

1¼ cups whole wheat flour
½ teaspoon baking soda
½ teaspoon baking powder
1½ teaspoons cinnamon
½ teaspoon kosher salt
1 cup quick cooking oats
½ cup unsweetened applesauce
3 tablespoons olive oil
2 large eggs, lightly beaten
⅓ cup unsweetened almond milk or 2% milk
1½ cups carrots, peeled and grated
1 cup zucchini, grated
1 ripe banana, mashed
2 tablespoons honey

Directions

1. Preheat oven to 400 degrees. Grease a 12-cup muffin pan or line with paper muffin cups.
2. Combine flour, baking soda, baking powder, cinnamon, salt and oats in a large bowl.
3. Combine applesauce, olive oil and eggs in a separate bowl; stir in milk, carrots, zucchini, banana and honey.
4. Add wet ingredients to flour mixture. Stir just until combined, making sure not to overmix.
5. Scoop mixture into muffin cups and bake until muffin tops begin to brown, about 20-25 minutes.
6. Cool for 10-15 minutes before eating.

Nutrition Facts

Zucchini-Carrot Muffins

Amount Per Serving

Calories 134	Calories from Fat 45

	% Daily Value*
Total Fat 5g	8%
Saturated Fat 1g	5%
Polyunsaturated Fat 1g	
Monounsaturated Fat 3g	
Cholesterol 15mg	5%
Sodium 138mg	6%
Potassium 171mg	5%
Total Carbohydrates 21g	7%
Dietary Fiber 3g	12%
Sugars 6g	
Protein 3g	6%
Vitamin A	47%
Vitamin C	14%
Calcium	3%
Iron	5%

* Percent Daily Values are based on a 2000 calorie diet.

Strawberry Mango Smoothie

Makes 4 servings

Make-Ahead Tip
Freeze single portions. Remove from freezer in the morning, pack it with your lunch and it should be thawed and ready shortly after you get to work.

Grab-and-Go Breakfast

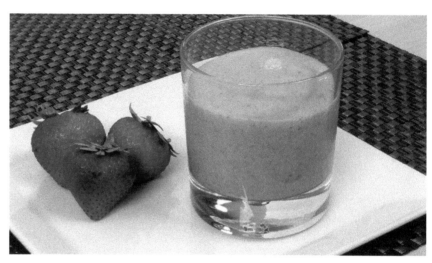

Ingredients

1 cup cold water
½ cup plain Greek yogurt, regular or low-fat
1½ cups frozen strawberries
1½ cups frozen mango
2 tablespoons honey
¼ cup ground flax seed
¼ teaspoon almond extract
1-2 scoops whey or vegetable protein powder (optional)

Directions

1. Pulse all ingredients in a blender until smooth.

Nutrition Facts
Strawberry Mango Smoothie

Amount Per Serving

Calories 124	Calories from Fat 36

	% Daily Value*
Total Fat 4g	6%
Polyunsaturated Fat 2g	
Monounsaturated Fat 1g	
Cholesterol 1mg	0%
Sodium 11mg	0%
Potassium 123mg	4%
Total Carbohydrates 23g	8%
Dietary Fiber 4g	16%
Sugars 10g	
Protein 7g	14%
Vitamin A	8%
Vitamin C	60%
Calcium	6%
Iron	4%

* Percent Daily Values are based on a 2000 calorie diet.

Banana Chocolate Smoothie with Flax Seed

Makes 4 servings

Make-Ahead Tip
Freeze single portions. Remove from freezer in the morning, pack it with your lunch and it should be thawed and ready shortly after you get to work.

Grab-and-Go Breakfast

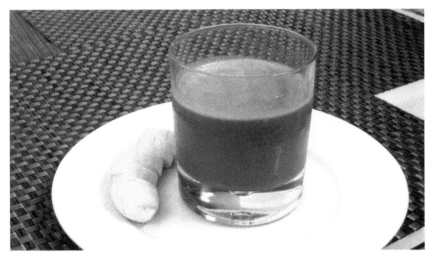

Ingredients

2 large bananas, about 2 cups
1 cup plain Greek yogurt, regular or low-fat
1 ½ cups 2% milk
1 teaspoon honey, optional, or to taste
3 tablespoons unsweetened cocoa powder
¼ cup ground flax seed
6 ice cubes

Directions

1. Place all ingredients in a blender and pulse until smooth and frothy.

Nutrition Facts
Banana Chocolate Flax Seed Smoothie

Amount Per Serving

Calories 186	Calories from Fat 45

	% Daily Value*
Total Fat 5g	8%
Saturated Fat 1g	5%
Polyunsaturated Fat 0.1g	
Monounsaturated Fat 1g	
Cholesterol 10mg	3%
Sodium 61mg	3%
Potassium 523mg	15%
Total Carbohydrates 28g	9%
Dietary Fiber 5g	20%
Sugars 16g	
Protein 23g	46%
Vitamin A	4%
Vitamin C	10%
Calcium	20%
Iron	6%

* Percent Daily Values are based on a 2000 calorie diet.

Lunch

Lunch should be one of your largest meals, since you need to renew your energy for the rest of the day. Foods available at work or school are frequently not good choices, so improve your nutrition and save some money by bringing food from home. This is easier if you have a refrigerator and microwave available at work, but a cold pack and a Thermos® will keep foods at safe and appetizing temperatures.

Batch cooking and packaging in lunch-sized portions can ease the planning process during the week and cooking extra portions of dinner entrées and bringing them for lunch is another easy solution for lunchtime nutrition.

Asian Chicken Cabbage Salad

Makes 6 servings

Make-Ahead Tip
Chicken can be cooked in advance and refrigerated or frozen.

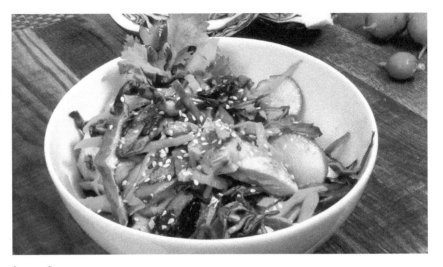

Nutrition Facts
Asian Chicken Cabbage Salad

Amount Per Serving

Calories 174	Calories from Fat 27
	% Daily Value*
Total Fat 3g	5%
Saturated Fat 0.3g	2%
Polyunsaturated Fat 0.3g	
Monounsaturated Fat 2g	
Cholesterol 65mg	22%
Sodium 140mg	6%
Potassium 513mg	15%
Total Carbohydrates 8g	3%
Dietary Fiber 2g	8%
Sugars 4g	
Protein 27g	54%
Vitamin A	136%
Vitamin C	53%
Calcium	4%
Iron	3%

* Percent Daily Values are based on a 2000 calorie diet.

Ingredients
24 ounces boneless, skinless chicken breast
1 tablespoon olive oil
1/4 teaspoon kosher salt
1/4 teaspoon black pepper
4 cups (about 1/2 head) red cabbage, shredded
2 cups shredded carrots
1/2 cup radishes, thinly sliced
1/4 cup green onion, cut on the bias in thin slices
1/4 cup cilantro, chopped
Juice of 1/2 fresh lime, or to taste
1/2 cup Asian vinaigrette dressing (page 67)
2 teaspoons sesame seeds, toasted, optional

Directions
1. Heat oil in skillet on medium-high heat.
2. Season chicken with salt and pepper. Cook chicken until browned on both sides, about 3-4 minutes per side.
3. Lower temperature to medium, cover and cook until chicken is tender and reaches an internal temperature of 165 degrees, about 8-10 additional minutes.
4. Cool chicken and chop into bite-sized pieces. Combine chicken, cabbage, carrots, radishes, onions and cilantro and toss with the Asian vinaigrette. Marinate at room temperature for at least 15-20 minutes, stirring occasionally.
5. To serve, drizzle lime juice over the salad and top with sesame seeds.

Greek Jar Salad

Makes 2 large or 4 small servings

Make-Ahead Tip
This salad will keep several days in the refrigerator with the dressing in the bottom of the jar.

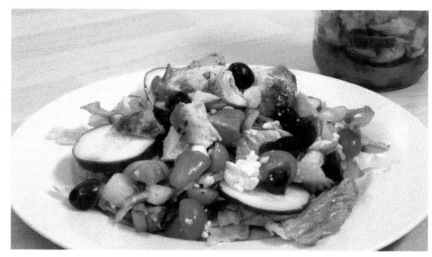

Ingredients
2 cups cherry tomatoes, quartered
2 cups cucumber, peeled and sliced
¼ cup red onion, diced
4 cups romaine lettuce, chopped
¼ cup Kalamata olives, pitted and halved
1 cup feta cheese, crumbled
2 cups cooked chicken, chopped
2 quart-size canning jars with lids

Directions
1. Make Citrus Vinaigrette recipe (page 67). Place about ¼ cup of the dressing in bottom of two 1-quart Mason jars and add cherry tomatoes.
2. Layer cucumber slices, followed by red onion and romaine lettuce, making sure to pack them down firmly in each jar.
3. Top off with Kalamata olives, feta cheese and chicken. Seal jars and refrigerate until ready to eat.
4. To serve, tilt and rotate jar to mix vinaigrette with salad, unscrew cap and place salad in serving dish of choice.

Nutrition Facts
Greek Jar Salad

Amount Per Serving	
Calories 202	Calories from Fat 72

	% Daily Value*
Total Fat 8g	**12%**
Saturated Fat 2g	**10%**
Trans Fat 0.01g	
Polyunsaturated Fat 0.3g	
Monounsaturated Fat 1g	
Cholesterol 49mg	**16%**
Sodium 495mg	**21%**
Potassium 460mg	**13%**
Total Carbohydrates 11g	**4%**
Dietary Fiber 6g	**24%**
Sugars 4g	
Protein 20g	**40%**
Vitamin A	116%
Vitamin C	57%
Calcium	7%
Iron	9%

* Percent Daily Values are based on a 2000 calorie diet.

Paprika Shrimp Spinach Salad

Makes 4 servings

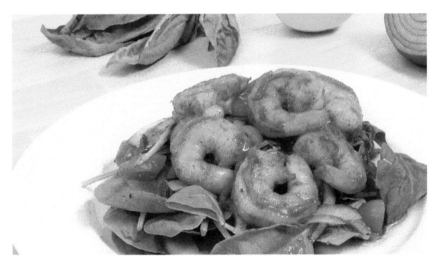

Ingredients

1½ pounds cooked shrimp, 16-20 count, peeled and deveined
  (if frozen, thaw and dry with paper towel)
6 tablespoons olive oil, divided
½ teaspoon paprika
¼ teaspoon kosher salt, divided
Zest of one lemon
5 ounces spinach (1 package)
1 large tomato, chopped
½ cup red onion, thinly sliced
2 tablespoons lemon juice
⅓ cup basil leaves, thinly sliced

Nutrition Facts

Paprika Shrimp Spinach Salad

Amount Per Serving

Calories 364	Calories from Fat 207

	% Daily Value*
Total Fat 23g	35%
Saturated Fat 3g	15%
Polyunsaturated Fat 23g	
Monounsaturated Fat 15g	
Cholesterol 330mg	110%
Sodium 480mg	20%
Potassium 358mg	10%
Total Carbohydrates 5g	2%
Dietary Fiber 2g	8%
Sugars 2g	
Protein 38g	76%
Vitamin A	83%
Vitamin C	36%
Calcium	10%
Iron	37%

* Percent Daily Values are based on a 2000 calorie diet.

Directions

1. In a bowl, combine shrimp with 1 tablespoon of olive oil, paprika, ⅛ teaspoon salt and lemon zest.
2. Heat a large skillet on medium heat, add shrimp and cook until warm and fragrant, stirring continuously, about 1-2 minutes. Remove from heat and set aside.
3. Toss spinach, tomatoes and onions in a bowl.
4. Combine remaining olive oil, lemon juice, basil and salt.
5. Pour dressing over salad and top with shrimp.
6. Dressed salad may also be portioned among four plates and topped with shrimp.

Tuna Avocado Salad

Makes 4 servings

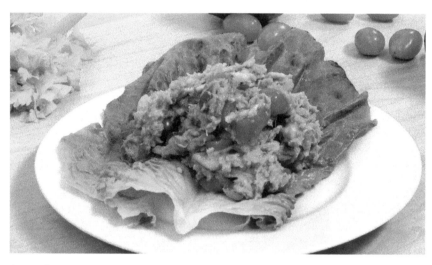

Ingredients

2 cans (6 oz.) water-packed tuna, drained
1 avocado, mashed
1 cup celery, chopped
$\frac{1}{3}$ cup red onion, chopped
3 tablespoons lemon juice
1 cup cherry or grape tomatoes, chopped
$\frac{1}{8}$ teaspoon salt
$\frac{1}{4}$ teaspoon black pepper
Romaine lettuce for plating (optional)

Directions

1. Combine all ingredients in a bowl.
2. Serve on top of salad greens or enjoy as a sandwich filling.

Nutrition Facts

Tuna Avocado Salad

Amount Per Serving

Calories 194	Calories from Fat 72

	% Daily Value*
Total Fat 8g	12%
Saturated Fat 1g	5%
Polyunsaturated Fat 1g	
Monounsaturated Fat 5g	
Cholesterol 25mg	8%
Sodium 343mg	14%
Potassium 617mg	18%
Total Carbohydrates 8g	3%
Dietary Fiber 4g	16%
Sugars 2g	
Protein 23g	46%
Vitamin A	11%
Vitamin C	24%
Calcium	3%
Iron	10%

* Percent Daily Values are based on a 2000 calorie diet.

Tomato Feta Quinoa Salad

Makes 8 servings

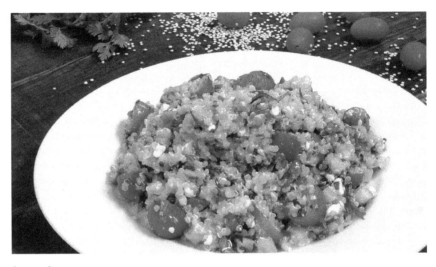

Ingredients

2 cups dry quinoa
4 cups water or low-sodium broth of choice
1 cup green onions, thinly sliced (include green parts)
1 cup fresh parsley, chopped
2 cups tomatoes, chopped
⅔ cup feta cheese, crumbled
½ cup extra virgin olive oil
⅔ cup fresh lemon juice

Directions

1. Cook quinoa according to package directions, with either water or broth. Cool. This may be done in advance.
2. Combine cooked quinoa, green onions, parsley, tomatoes and cheese.
3. Drizzle with olive oil and lemon juice and toss.
4. This salad is delicious served hot or cold.

Nutrition Facts

Tomato Feta Quinoa Salad

Amount Per Serving

Calories 328	Calories from Fat 162

	% Daily Value*
Total Fat 18g	**28%**
Saturated Fat 3g	**15%**
Polyunsaturated Fat 1g	
Monounsaturated Fat 10g	
Cholesterol 6mg	**2%**
Sodium 192mg	**8%**
Potassium 208mg	**6%**
Total Carbohydrates 36g	**12%**
Dietary Fiber 5g	**20%**
Sugars 3g	
Protein 8g	**16%**
Vitamin A	24%
Vitamin C	45%
Calcium	7%
Iron	26%

* Percent Daily Values are based on a 2000 calorie diet.

Southwestern Bean Salad

Makes 8 servings

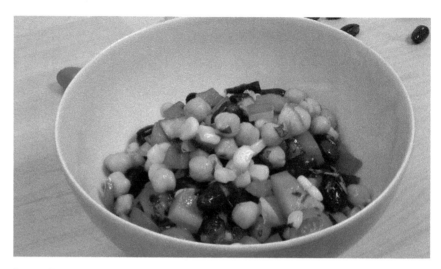

Ingredients

2 15-ounce cans low-sodium garbanzo beans, rinsed and drained
2 15-ounce cans low-sodium kidney beans, rinsed and drained
3 cups red bell pepper, diced
1 cup red onion, diced
2 cups cherry tomatoes, halved
2 cups frozen corn, thawed
½ cup cilantro, minced
2 jalapeño peppers, seeded and finely diced (optional)
½ cup lime juice
½ cup extra virgin olive oil

Directions

1. In large bowl, combine all ingredients except lime juice and olive oil.
2. Combine lime juice and olive oil; pour over salad and toss to evenly coat salad.

Nutrition Facts
Southwestern Bean Salad

Amount Per Serving

Calories 397	Calories from Fat 153

	% Daily Value*
Total Fat 17g	26%
Saturated Fat 2g	10%
Polyunsaturated Fat 2g	
Monounsaturated Fat 10g	
Sodium 172mg	7%
Potassium 370mg	11%
Total Carbohydrates 45g	15%
Dietary Fiber 17g	68%
Sugars 6g	
Protein 16g	32%
Vitamin A	45%
Vitamin C	202%
Calcium	10%
Iron	21%

* Percent Daily Values are based on a 2000 calorie diet.

Chicken BLT Wraps

Makes 4 servings

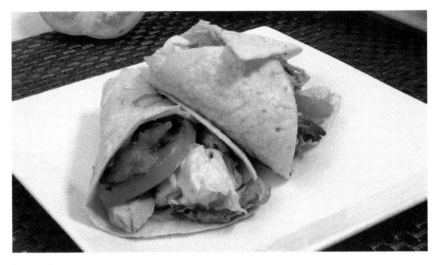

Ingredients

1 pound boneless, skinless chicken breast
1 tablespoon olive oil
¼ teaspoon kosher salt
¼ teaspoon black pepper
8 large Bibb lettuce leaves, or other salad greens
8 slices bacon, cooked
2 large ripe tomatoes, sliced
1 avocado, sliced
4 whole wheat tortillas
1 cup Lemon Cumin Yogurt Sauce (page 70)

Directions

1. Heat a large sauté pan on medium-high heat and add olive oil.
2. Season chicken with salt and pepper and place in pan.
3. Cook chicken until browned on one side, about 3-4 minutes. Flip and brown on other side, another 3-4 minutes.
4. Cover and cook until chicken is tender and reaches an internal temperature of 165 degrees, about 8-10 additional minutes.
5. Cool chicken and chop into bite-sized pieces. This can be prepared in advance, and held in the refrigerator, or frozen and thawed when ready to use.
6. Coat chopped chicken pieces with Lemon Cumin Yogurt Sauce.
7. Build wraps with tortilla on bottom layer, followed by lettuce and chicken. Top with bacon, tomatoes and avocado. Roll tightly and cut in half to serve.

Nutrition Facts

Chicken BLT Wraps

Amount Per Serving

Calories 471	Calories from Fat 189

	% Daily Value*
Total Fat 21g	32%
Saturated Fat 4g	20%
Polyunsaturated Fat 1g	
Monounsaturated Fat 7g	
Cholesterol 96mg	32%
Sodium 543mg	23%
Potassium 833mg	24%
Total Carbohydrates 34g	11%
Dietary Fiber 8g	32%
Sugars 4g	
Protein 43g	86%
Vitamin A	37%
Vitamin C	30%
Calcium	2%
Iron	15%

* Percent Daily Values are based on a 2000 calorie diet.

Savory Turkey Wrap

Makes 4 servings

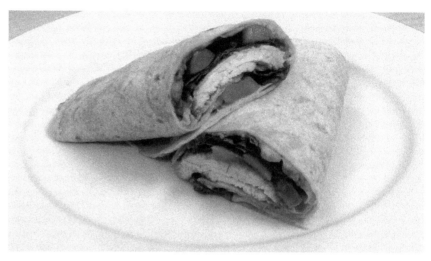

Ingredients

4 12-inch whole grain tortillas
½ cup hummus
½ cup guacamole
¾ cup red bell pepper, diced
½ cup green onions, thinly sliced (include green parts)
8 ounces cooked turkey, deli-style is fine
1 cup fresh spinach, chopped
¼ cup store-bought salsa (low-sodium, no added sugar)

Directions

1. Lay out tortillas on a flat surface.
2. Spread hummus and guacamole evenly on tortillas.
3. Add peppers and onions, spreading evenly.
4. Add turkey, spinach and salsa.
5. Roll up, cut in half and serve.
6. If serving as an appetizer or snack, cut into medallions.

Nutrition Facts

Savory Turkey Wrap

Amount Per Serving

Calories 292	Calories from Fat 108

	% Daily Value*
Total Fat 12g	18%
Saturated Fat 2g	10%
Polyunsaturated Fat 3g	
Monounsaturated Fat 6g	
Cholesterol 30mg	10%
Sodium 347mg	14%
Potassium 573mg	16%
Total Carbohydrates 29g	10%
Dietary Fiber 7g	28%
Sugars 3g	
Protein 18g	36%
Vitamin A	37%
Vitamin C	105%
Calcium	4%
Iron	14%

* Percent Daily Values are based on a 2000 calorie diet.

Penne with Sausage & Kale

Makes 6 servings

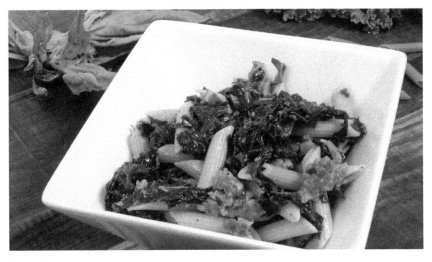

Ingredients

½ pound dry whole grain penne pasta
1 tablespoon olive oil
¾ pound spicy ground Italian sausage
2 tablespoons garlic, minced
½ cup yellow onion, chopped
¾ cup water, divided
2 tablespoons butter
2 tablespoons fresh lemon juice
6 cups fresh baby kale, chopped thinly
¼ teaspoon salt
½ teaspoon black pepper

Directions

1. Cook pasta according to package directions and drain.
2. Preheat a large sauté pan on medium-high heat. Add olive oil and sausage to pan and cook through, breaking sausage into small pieces.
3. Reduce heat to medium. Add kale, garlic and onions; cover and cook until kale is tender, about 12-15 minutes. Stir periodically.
4. Add cooked pasta, butter, lemon juice, basil, salt and pepper, mix well. Cover and cook on low for about 5 minutes.

Nutrition Facts

Penne with Italian Sausage and Kale

Amount Per Serving

Calories 397	Calories from Fat 225

	% Daily Value*
Total Fat 25g	**38%**
Saturated Fat 9g	**45%**
Polyunsaturated Fat 3g	
Monounsaturated Fat 11g	
Cholesterol 54mg	**18%**
Sodium 505mg	**21%**
Potassium 176mg	**5%**
Total Carbohydrates 31g	**10%**
Dietary Fiber 5g	**20%**
Sugars 2g	
Protein 15g	**30%**
Vitamin A	12%
Vitamin C	63%
Calcium	8%
Iron	7%

* Percent Daily Values are based on a 2000 calorie diet.

Tuscan Bean Soup

Makes 8 servings

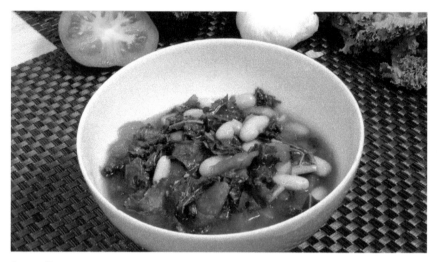

Ingredients

½ cup olive oil

8 cups kale, about 2 bunches, washed and thinly sliced or chopped

½ teaspoon kosher salt

½ teaspoon black pepper

2 14.5-ounce cans diced tomatoes

4 cups vegetable or chicken broth

2 15-ounce cans low-sodium cannellini beans, rinsed and drained

2 teaspoons garlic, minced

Directions

1. Heat olive oil in a soup pot on medium-high heat.
2. Add kale, salt and pepper; stir and cook 1-2 minutes.
3. Add tomatoes, broth and beans.
4. Bring to a boil; reduce heat to a simmer.
5. Cover and simmer for 30 minutes or until kale is tender.
6. Stir in garlic and remove from heat.
7. Makes about 10 cups.

Nutrition Facts

Tuscan Bean Soup

Amount Per Serving

Calories 261	Calories from Fat 126

	% Daily Value*
Total Fat 14g	22%
Saturated Fat 2g	10%
Polyunsaturated Fat 2g	
Monounsaturated Fat 10g	
Sodium 402mg	17%
Potassium 876mg	25%
Total Carbohydrates 28g	9%
Dietary Fiber 8g	32%
Sugars 3g	
Protein 15g	30%
Vitamin A	209%
Vitamin C	177%
Calcium	20%
Iron	21%

* Percent Daily Values are based on a 2000 calorie diet.

Snacks

Plan on making snacks at home, since good snack choices are hard to find at work or school. Eat them for your mid-morning and mid-afternoon re-fueling. Prepare our recipes or grab simple ready-to-eat options like fruits, vegetables, nuts/seeds or cheese. Snack bars should be a last resort, but it may be smart to keep a few low-sugar (not artificially sweetened) snack bars in your desk drawer in case you forget to bring snacks from home.

Oat Chocolate Crumble Bars

Makes 16 bars

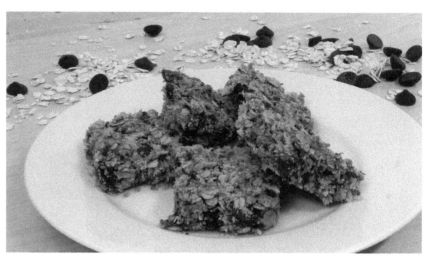

Ingredients

1¼ cups old-fashioned rolled oats
¼ cup oat flour or finely ground rolled oats
¾ cup unsweetened flaked coconut
⅓ cup dry quinoa, cooked according to package directions
¼ teaspoon kosher salt
¼ teaspoon cinnamon
1 cup dark chocolate chips
¼ cup creamy almond butter or peanut butter
¼ cup water

Directions

1. Preheat oven to 350 degrees. Grease an 8x8-inch baking pan.
2. Combine oats, oat flour, coconut, quinoa, salt, cinnamon and chocolate chips in a large mixing bowl.
3. Add the almond butter (or peanut butter) and water and mix well.
4. Firmly press mixture into pan using the bottom of a glass or a large spoon. Mixture will be 1 inch thick.
5. Bake until golden brown, about 30-35 minutes.
6. Cool completely before cutting with a sharp knife.

Nutrition Facts

Oat Chocolate Crumble Bars

Amount Per Serving

Calories 156	Calories from Fat 81

	% Daily Value*
Total Fat 9g	14%
Saturated Fat 5g	25%
Polyunsaturated Fat 0.5g	
Monounsaturated Fat 2g	
Sodium 42mg	2%
Potassium 35mg	1%
Total Carbohydrates 18g	6%
Dietary Fiber 3g	12%
Sugars 9g	
Protein 3g	6%
Vitamin C	0.02%
Calcium	2%
Iron	11%

* Percent Daily Values are based on a 2000 calorie diet.

Sweet and Savory Energy Bites

Makes 16

Make-Ahead Tip
Store in an airtight container, refrigerated, for up to 1 week. Make in large batches and freeze for months.

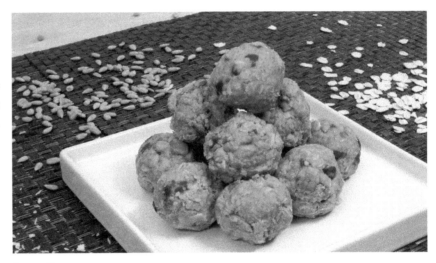

Ingredients
1 cup old-fashioned rolled oats
⅔ cup creamy peanut butter, or other nut butter
½ cup unsweetened coconut flakes
¼ cup ground flax seed
¼ cup mini dark chocolate chips
¼ cup sunflower seeds
1 teaspoon almond extract
½ teaspoon cinnamon
¼ teaspoon kosher salt

Directions
1. Thoroughly mix all ingredients together in a medium bowl.
2. Roll into firmly packed golf ball-sized balls, about two tablespoons each. These taste even better the next day, after the flavors blend.

Nutrition Facts
Sweet and Savory Energy Bites

Amount Per Serving

Calories 129	Calories from Fat 81

	% Daily Value*
Total Fat 9g	14%
Saturated Fat 3g	15%
Polyunsaturated Fat 1g	
Monounsaturated Fat 0.3g	
Sodium 60mg	3%
Potassium 18mg	1%
Total Carbohydrates 10g	3%
Dietary Fiber 2g	8%
Sugars 3g	
Protein 4g	8%
Vitamin C	0.03%
Calcium	1%
Iron	4%

* Percent Daily Values are based on a 2000 calorie diet.

Cannellini Bean Dip

Makes 6 ⅓-cup servings

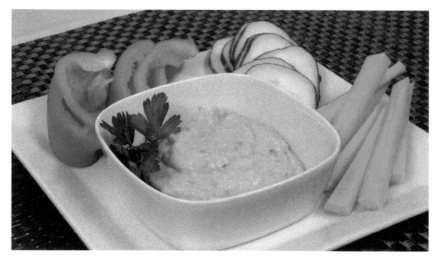

Ingredients

¼ cup olive oil
2 15-ounce cans low-sodium cannellini beans,
    rinsed and drained
1 tablespoon garlic
1 tablespoon fresh rosemary, minced
2 tablespoons lemon juice
¼ teaspoon kosher salt
⅛ teaspoon black pepper
¼ cup water

Directions

1. In a blender, combine olive oil, beans, garlic, rosemary, lemon juice, and salt and pepper.
2. Blend until smooth, adding just enough water to keep the blender moving, about ¼ cup.
3. Serve with vegetables, pita chips or crackers.

Nutrition Facts
Cannellini Bean Dip

Amount Per Serving

Calories 182	Calories from Fat 81
	% Daily Value*
Total Fat 9g	14%
Saturated Fat 1g	5%
Polyunsaturated Fat 1g	
Monounsaturated Fat 7g	
Sodium 157mg	7%
Potassium 8mg	0%
Total Carbohydrates 20g	7%
Dietary Fiber 7g	28%
Sugars 0.02g	
Protein 6g	12%
Vitamin A	0.2%
Vitamin C	3%
Calcium	4%
Iron	11%

* Percent Daily Values are based on a 2000 calorie diet.

Creamy Spicy Bean Dip

Makes 9 ⅓-cup servings

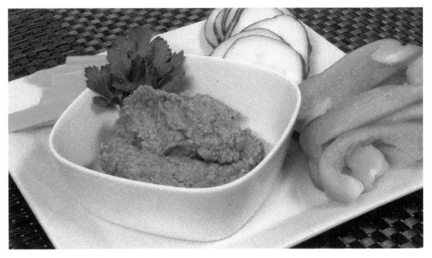

Ingredients

¼ cup olive oil
½ teaspoon garlic, powder or granulated
¼ cup red onion, diced
2 teaspoons chili powder
2 teaspoons cumin
½ teaspoon dried basil
1 15-ounce can low-sodium black beans, rinsed and drained
1 15-ounce can low-sodium garbanzo beans, rinsed and drained
2 tablespoons fresh lime juice (about 1 lime)
¼ cup water
½ teaspoon salt
1 teaspoon Tabasco or sriracha sauce, or to taste

Directions

1. Place all ingredients in a blender or food processor and blend until smooth.
2. Serve with vegetables, crackers or chips.

Nutrition Facts

Creamy Spicy Bean Dip

Amount Per Serving

Calories 199	Calories from Fat 99

	% Daily Value*
Total Fat 11g	17%
Saturated Fat 1g	5%
Polyunsaturated Fat 2g	
Monounsaturated Fat 13g	
Sodium 279mg	12%
Potassium 48mg	1%
Total Carbohydrates 21g	7%
Dietary Fiber 7g	28%
Sugars 1g	
Protein 7g	14%
Vitamin A	5%
Vitamin C	5%
Calcium	4%
Iron	10%

* Percent Daily Values are based on a 2000 calorie diet.

Roasted Edamame

Makes 8 ¼-cup servings

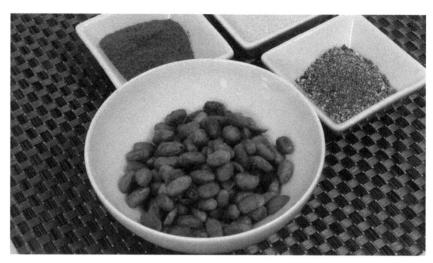

Ingredients

1 20-ounce package frozen shelled edamame (soybeans), thawed
¼ cup olive oil
1 teaspoon garlic powder
1 teaspoon paprika
½ teaspoon salt
¼ teaspoon black pepper

Directions

1. Preheat oven to 400 degrees. Line a baking sheet with foil or parchment paper.
2. Mix together olive oil, garlic powder, paprika, salt and pepper in a bowl.
3. Add edamame beans to the bowl and toss gently, making sure beans are evenly coated.
4. Place beans on baking sheet in a single layer. Roast for 10-15 minutes until beans start to brown.
5. Raise oven temperature to broil and cook edamame until lightly brown, an additional 5-7 minutes.
6. Cool completely and package in individual snack bags.

Nutrition Facts

Roasted Edamame

Amount Per Serving

Calories 123	Calories from Fat 81
	% Daily Value*
Total Fat 9g	14%
Saturated Fat 1g	5%
Polyunsaturated Fat 1g	
Monounsaturated Fat 10g	
Sodium 149mg	6%
Potassium 263mg	8%
Total Carbohydrates 5g	2%
Dietary Fiber 3g	12%
Sugars 1g	
Protein 6g	12%
Vitamin A	3%
Vitamin C	10%
Calcium	4%
Iron	7%

* Percent Daily Values are based on a 2000 calorie diet.

Turkey Wild Rice Meatballs

Makes 4 servings

Make-Ahead Tip
Recipe may be doubled and frozen.

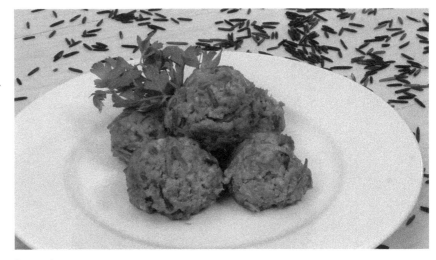

Ingredients

½ cup dry wild rice
1 pound ground turkey
1 large egg, slightly beaten
½ cup red onion, finely chopped
½ teaspoon ground turmeric
1 teaspoon ground paprika
1 teaspoon ground cumin
2 tablespoons minced garlic
2 tablespoons fresh lime juice (about 1 lime)
½ teaspoon salt

Directions

1. Cook wild rice according to package directions. This can be done in advance.
2. Preheat oven to 400 degrees. Line a baking sheet with foil or parchment paper.
3. Combine all ingredients and mix thoroughly.
4. Shape into 16 balls and place on baking sheet.
5. Bake until lightly browned and firm to the touch, about 15-20 minutes.

Nutrition Facts

Turkey-Wild Rice Meatballs

Amount Per Serving

Calories 279	Calories from Fat 99

	% Daily Value*
Total Fat 11g	17%
Saturated Fat 3g	15%
Trans Fat 0.3g	
Polyunsaturated Fat 3g	
Monounsaturated Fat 4g	
Cholesterol 143mg	48%
Sodium 419mg	17%
Potassium 447mg	13%
Total Carbohydrates 20g	7%
Dietary Fiber 2g	8%
Sugars 2g	
Protein 25g	50%
Vitamin A	7%
Vitamin C	11%
Calcium	5%
Iron	15%

* Percent Daily Values are based on a 2000 calorie diet.

Trail Mix

Makes 14 ¼-cup servings

Make-Ahead Tip
Pack trail mix in single-serving resealable bags.

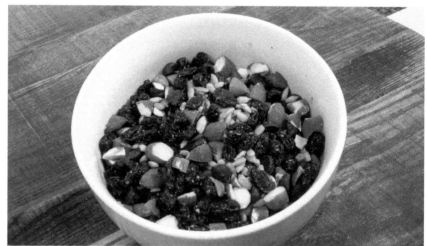

Ingredients

1 cup raisins
1 cup almonds, or other nut of choice, chopped if desired
1 cup sunflower seeds, salted if desired
½ cup dark chocolate chips

Directions

1. Combine ingredients.

Nutrition Facts

Trail Mix

Amount Per Serving

Calories 211	Calories from Fat 126

	% Daily Value*
Total Fat 14g	**22%**
Saturated Fat 3g	**15%**
Polyunsaturated Fat 5g	
Monounsaturated Fat 5g	
Sodium 62mg	**3%**
Potassium 245mg	**7%**
Total Carbohydrates 18g	**6%**
Dietary Fiber 3g	**12%**
Sugars 6g	
Protein 6g	**12%**
Vitamin C	0.3%
Calcium	4%
Iron	6%

* Percent Daily Values are based on a 2000 calorie diet.

Banana Nut Energy Bites

Makes 12 servings

Make-Ahead Tip
Layer Energy Bites between waxed paper in an airtight container. Store in refrigerator up to 3 days or freeze up to 3 months.

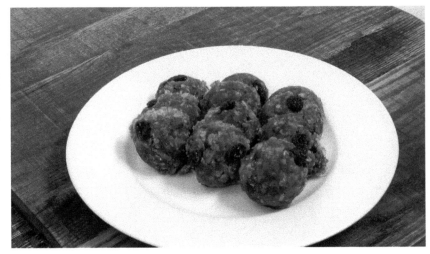

Ingredients
1 large overripe banana
1 cup dry quick-cooking rolled oats
½ cup sunflower seeds
⅓ cup raisins
¾ cup natural creamy peanut butter (no sugar added)
¼ cup dark mini chocolate chips

Directions
1. In a medium bowl, mash banana with a fork until smooth. Stir in oats, sunflower seeds, raisins, peanut butter and chocolate chips.
2. Roll into tablespoon-sized balls and flatten slightly for 24 pieces. Or, combine two tablespoons into larger balls for 12 pieces.

Nutrition Facts
Banana Nut Energy Snacks

Amount Per Serving

Calories 207	Calories from Fat 108

	% Daily Value*
Total Fat 12g	18%
Saturated Fat 2g	10%
Polyunsaturated Fat 2g	
Monounsaturated Fat 1g	
Sodium 29mg	1%
Potassium 71mg	2%
Total Carbohydrates 18g	6%
Dietary Fiber 3g	12%
Sugars 7g	
Protein 7g	14%
Vitamin A	0.2%
Vitamin C	2%
Calcium	2%
Iron	4%

* Percent Daily Values are based on a 2000 calorie diet.

Quick & Easy Snack Ideas

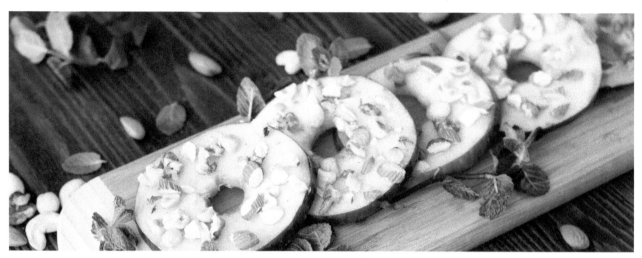

Snacks can be very simple and easy to prepare. The trick is to do some planning so you (and your children) have snack foods available. This enables eating frequently enough to maintain a high energy level and keep your blood sugar stable so you are not tempted to overeat sugary and salty foods.

Following are several tips and ideas for simple but satisfying snacks, courtesy of the USDA and the Chef Marshall O'Brien Group:

Make it a combo

Combine food groups for satisfying snacks that supply lean protein, healthy fats and slow carbohydrates. These three macronutrients should be part of every meal and snack to provide you with great energy and stable blood sugar.

Eat vibrant veggies

Brightly colored vegetables contain a wide variety of nutrients. To tempt taste buds, spice up raw vegetables with dips that contain the healthy fat needed to absorb fat-soluble nutrients. Try dipping bell peppers, carrots, or cucumbers in hummus, tzatziki, guacamole, or a homemade ranch dressing. Cut up some extra veggies when you are preparing dinner so you always have them on hand.

Build your own snack mix

Make your own high-quality trail mix with unsalted nuts and add-ins such as sunflower or pumpkin seeds, dried fruit, popcorn, or a sprinkle of chocolate chips.

Prep ahead for grab-and-go convenience

Portion snack foods into baggies or containers when you get home from the store so they're ready to go when you need them. This also helps with portion control: Some tasty, healthy snacks are high in calories, so they should be consumed in controlled quantities.

Snack on the go

Take ready-to-eat snacks when you're out. A banana (or apple or orange), yogurt (in a cooler), or baby carrots are delicious, portable and provide essential nutrients.

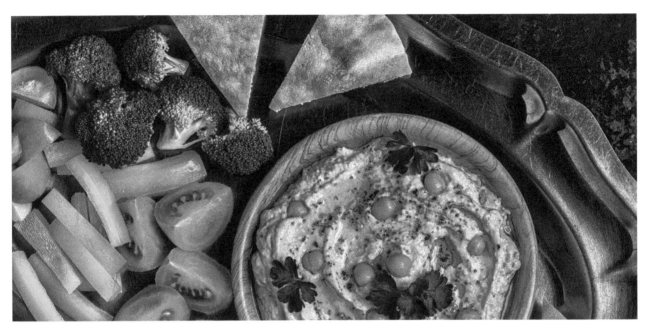

Simple Snack Ideas

Smoothies

Blend plain yogurt with 100% fruit juice and frozen peaches for a tasty smoothie. Prepare and freeze individual servings the night before and they will be thawed by the time you need a mid-morning snack.

Yogurt

Mix fresh or frozen fruit with plain yogurt for an easy, satisfying snack.

Nibble on lean protein

Choose lean protein foods such as low-sodium, nitrate-free deli meats or unsalted nuts. Wrap sliced, low-sodium deli turkey around an apple wedge. Store hard-cooked (boiled) eggs in the refrigerator for kids to enjoy any time.

Don't forget the healthy fat

Healthy fats such as butter, cream cheese, avocado and nut butter help you absorb fat-soluble vitamins such as A, D, E and K. They also help stabilize blood sugar by slowing the absorption of carbohydrates and contribute to the feeling of satiety.

Snacks such as celery sticks with cream cheese or nut butter, apples with nut butter and nitrate-free deli meat roll-ups spread with cream cheese are tasty and satisfying.

Focus on whole grains

Pair whole grain crackers with nitrate-free deli meats or cheese; use whole grain tortillas as the base for turkey, avocado, and salsa roll-ups. Limit refined-grain products such as snack bars, cakes, and sweetened cereals.

Fruits are quick and easy

Fresh fruits can be easy "grab-and-go" options that need little preparation and keep well.

Consider convenience

A single-serving container of low-fat yogurt or individually wrapped string cheese can be just enough for an after-school snack.

Homemade goodies reduce sugar

For homemade sweets, add dried fruits like apricots or raisins and reduce the amount of sugar in the recipe. Adjust recipes that include fats like butter by using unsweetened apple-sauce to reduce the fat.

Dinner

We all come home tired and hungry and, if we don't have a quick and easy solution for dinner, we will likely eat the wrong things. So we created dinner recipes that can be made in 30 minutes or less.

In addition, consider this: Dinner should not be your biggest meal of the day. Most people are less active in the evening, so they need fewer calories later in the day. Remember that when you eat, you either burn the calories as energy or wear them as fat. If your activity level is low in the evening, make dinner a smaller meal.

One Pan Mediterranean Chicken

Makes 8 servings

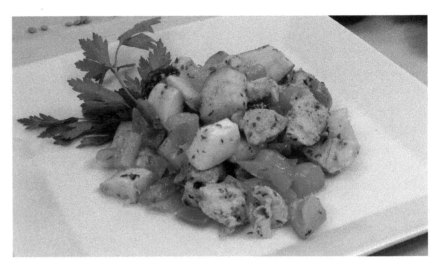

Ingredients

3 pounds chicken breast, chopped in bite-sized pieces

6 cups red bell pepper, in large chunks

8 cups zucchini or yellow summer squash, in large chunks

2 cups red onion, chopped in large chunks

½ cup olive oil

¼ cup honey

½ cup lemon juice

2 teaspoons dried parsley

2 teaspoons dried thyme

2 teaspoons dried oregano

½ teaspoon salt

½ teaspoon black pepper

4 cups cooked brown rice or quinoa, optional

Directions

1. Preheat oven to 350 degrees. Line a sheet pan with foil or parchment paper.
2. Place chicken and vegetables in a bowl. Drizzle with olive oil, honey and lemon juice; then sprinkle with spices. Toss together thoroughly and transfer to sheet pan.
3. Bake 20-25 minutes, or until chicken reaches an internal temperature of 165 degrees.
4. Serve over rice or quinoa, if desired.

Nutrition Facts

One-Pan Mediterranean Chicken

Amount Per Serving

Calories 374	Calories from Fat 144

	% Daily Value*
Total Fat 16g	25%
Saturated Fat 2g	10%
Polyunsaturated Fat 2g	
Monounsaturated Fat 10g	
Cholesterol 90mg	30%
Sodium 231mg	10%
Potassium 984mg	28%
Total Carbohydrates 20g	7%
Dietary Fiber 5g	20%
Sugars 13g	
Protein 39g	78%
Vitamin A	76%
Vitamin C	406%
Calcium	5%
Iron	9%

* Percent Daily Values are based on a 2000 calorie diet.

Turkey Bolognese Pasta

Makes 8 servings

Make-Ahead Tip
Pasta may be made in advance (undercook slightly) and stored in the refrigerator. To reheat, add pasta to a saucepan of boiling water and cook about 1 minute or until pasta is hot and tender. Drain well.

Cooking Definition
Deglazing a pan is done after meat has been browned and removed. Add water, broth or wine to the pan, scrape the browned bits off the bottom of the pan and stir to create a sauce or pan gravy.

Recommended Toppings
Grated Parmesan cheese

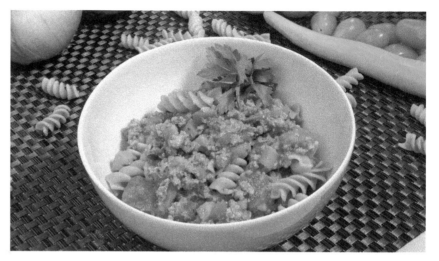

Ingredients
1 pound dry whole grain rotini pasta
2 pounds lean ground turkey
2 tablespoons olive oil
2 tablespoons garlic, minced
2 small white or yellow onions, diced
4 carrots, peeled and diced
¼ cup tomato paste
2 cups low-sodium chicken broth
2 28-ounce cans diced, no-salt-added tomatoes
4 bay leaves
1 teaspoon salt
1 teaspoon black pepper
1 cup Parmesan cheese, grated (optional)
Sprigs of fresh parsley (optional garnish)

Directions
1. Cook pasta according to package directions.
2. Heat oil in a large skillet on medium-high heat. Cook turkey, breaking up large pieces with a spatula or wooden spoon.
3. Add garlic, onion, carrots and bay leaves. Sauté until softened, about 3-5 minutes. Add tomato paste to bottom of pan; caramelize 3-5 minutes.
4. Deglaze pan with the broth, then stir in tomatoes, salt and pepper. Reduce heat to a simmer and cook until liquid is reduced by half, or about 25-30 minutes, stirring occasionally.
5. Remove bay leaves. Pour sauce over hot pasta and mix gently. Top with Parmesan cheese and garnish with parsley, as desired.

Nutrition Facts
Turkey Bolognese Pasta

Amount Per Serving

Calories 420	Calories from Fat 90
	% Daily Value*
Total Fat 10g	15%
Saturated Fat 3g	15%
Polyunsaturated Fat 0.4g	
Monounsaturated Fat 0.1g	
Cholesterol 65mg	22%
Sodium 286mg	12%
Potassium 555mg	16%
Total Carbohydrates 56g	19%
Dietary Fiber 3g	12%
Sugars 6g	
Protein 33g	66%
Vitamin A	112%
Vitamin C	32%
Calcium	8%
Iron	25%

* Percent Daily Values are based on a 2000 calorie diet.

Chicken & Pinto Beans

Makes 8 servings

Recommended Toppings
Chopped cilantro
Lime wedges

Make-Ahead Tip
Portion the meal into serving-sized containers and refrigerate for several days or freeze for several months.

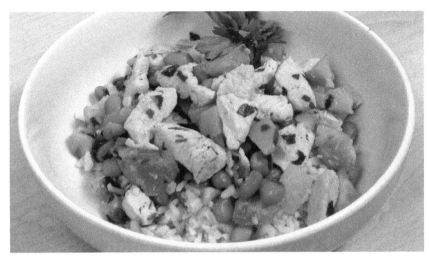

Nutrition Facts
Chicken and Pinto Beans

Amount Per Serving

Calories 236	Calories from Fat 36

	% Daily Value *
Total Fat 4g	7 %
Saturated Fat 0g	2 %
Monounsaturated Fat 2g	
Polyunsaturated Fat 0g	
Trans Fat 0g	
Cholesterol 55mg	18 %
Sodium 213mg	9 %
Potassium 120mg	3 %
Total Carbohydrates 37g	12 %
Dietary Fiber 23g	91 %
Sugars 3g	
Protein 35g	71 %
Vitamin A	51 %
Vitamin C	44 %
Calcium	15 %
Iron	28 %

*Percent Daily Values are based on a 2000 calorie diet

Ingredients

1 tablespoon olive oil
1 pound boneless, skinless chicken breast, cut in bite-sized pieces
$\frac{1}{4}$ teaspoon salt, or to taste
2 teaspoons garlic, minced
$\frac{1}{2}$ cup red bell pepper, diced
$1\frac{1}{2}$ cups pinto beans, rinsed and thoroughly drained
$\frac{1}{4}$ cup tomatoes, diced
$\frac{1}{4}$ cup fresh parsley, finely chopped
$\frac{1}{4}$ cup green onions, thinly sliced
2 tablespoons lime juice, or to taste (about 1 large)
$1\frac{1}{2}$ cups dry brown rice, optional
3 cups water or low-sodium broth, for cooking rice

Directions

1. Optional: if serving with rice, cook rice according to package directions and set aside.
2. Heat oil in skillet over medium heat. Add chicken and season with salt and pepper.
3. Cook chicken, stirring periodically, until almost firm to the touch—about 3 minutes.
4. Add garlic, bell peppers, beans and tomatoes, and mix well.
5. Continue cooking until chicken is fully cooked and mixture is heated through, about 2-3 minutes.
6. Add parsley, green onions and fresh lime juice; stir until incorporated. Adjust taste as desired.
7. Remove from heat, portion and serve.

Southwestern Chicken & Veggie Bake

Makes 4 servings

Make-Ahead Tip
Freeze chicken/vegetable mixture and rice separately in serving-sized containers. To serve, gently warm them on the stovetop or in the microwave.

Recommended Toppings
Chopped cilantro
Lime wedges
Hot sauce

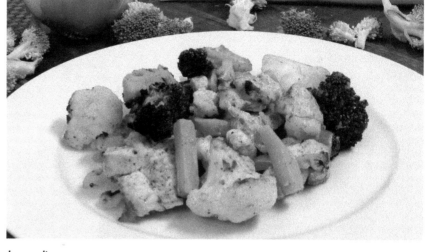

Ingredients
24 ounces boneless, skinless chicken breast, chopped small
2 16-ounce bags frozen California blend vegetables
   (broccoli, cauliflower and carrots)
1 cup onion, sliced
¼ cup olive oil
2 teaspoons paprika
2 teaspoons cumin
½ teaspoon garlic powder
¼ teaspoon kosher salt

Directions
1. Preheat oven to 350 degrees. Line a sheet pan with foil or parchment paper.
2. In a large bowl, mix together the chicken, vegetables and onions. Drizzle the olive oil and sprinkle spices over chicken and vegetables; mix well and spread on sheet pan.
3. Bake 20-25 minutes, or until chicken reaches an internal temperature of 165 degrees.
4. Serve over brown rice, quinoa or other whole grain. Add recommended toppings, as desired.

Nutrition Facts
Southwestern Chicken and Veggie Bake

Amount Per Serving

Calories 364	Calories from Fat 135

	% Daily Value*
Total Fat 15g	23%
Saturated Fat 2g	10%
Polyunsaturated Fat 2g	
Monounsaturated Fat 10g	
Cholesterol 98mg	33%
Sodium 184mg	8%
Potassium 648mg	19%
Total Carbohydrates 12g	4%
Dietary Fiber 3g	12%
Sugars 5g	
Protein 42g	84%
Vitamin A	37%
Vitamin C	40%
Calcium	6%
Iron	8%

* Percent Daily Values are based on a 2000 calorie diet.

Herbed Salmon Burgers

Makes 4 servings

Make-Ahead Tip

The patties may be made ahead. Freeze them uncooked to have them readily available for quick meals.

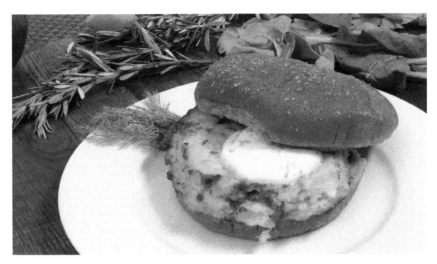

Ingredients

1¼ pounds wild-caught salmon, skin and fat line removed
1 large egg, beaten
½ cup bread crumbs
¼ cup red onion, minced
2 teaspoons fresh rosemary, minced
2 teaspoons Dijon mustard
¼ teaspoon kosher salt
¼ teaspoon black pepper
1 tablespoon olive oil, plus additional for basting
2 teaspoons lemon juice
4 whole wheat buns, optional
Lemon-Dill Sauce, page 70, optional

Directions

1. Cut salmon into long strips; mince in uniformly sized pieces.
2. In a large bowl, combine egg and bread crumbs; set aside until egg is absorbed into bread crumbs, about 5 minutes.
3. Add onion, rosemary, mustard, salt, black pepper, olive oil, and lemon juice; mix thoroughly.
4. Chill in refrigerator for at least 1 hour.
5. Portion salmon into four equal patties.
6. Brush remaining olive oil on both sides of patties; grill until the internal temperature reaches 145 degrees or desired doneness.
7. If desired, serve burgers on whole-wheat hamburger buns with Lemon Dill Sauce.

Nutrition Facts

Herbed Salmon Burgers

Amount Per Serving

Calories 271	Calories from Fat 99

	% Daily Value*
Total Fat 11g	17%
Saturated Fat 2g	10%
Polyunsaturated Fat 1g	
Monounsaturated Fat 3g	
Cholesterol 128mg	43%
Sodium 320mg	13%
Potassium 61mg	2%
Total Carbohydrates 12g	4%
Dietary Fiber 1g	4%
Sugars 1g	
Protein 31g	62%
Vitamin A	4%
Vitamin C	4%
Calcium	5%
Iron	8%

* Percent Daily Values are based on a 2000 calorie diet.

Balsamic Glazed Salmon with Asparagus

Makes 4 servings

Make-Ahead Tip
If you prefer to skin the salmon ahead of time, a bread knife works well for removing the skin. Otherwise, the skin is easy to remove after the salmon is cooked.

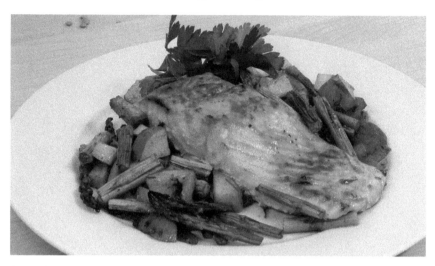

Ingredients

24 ounces salmon (4 6-ounce filets)
1 pound asparagus, cut in 1-inch pieces
1 pound baby red potatoes, cut in bite-sized pieces

Marinade Ingredients

2 tablespoons olive oil
1 tablespoon honey
3 tablespoons balsamic vinegar
1 tablespoon Dijon mustard
1 teaspoon fresh thyme, chopped
¼ teaspoon salt
¼ teaspoon black pepper

Directions

1. Preheat oven to 450 degrees. Line a sheet pan with foil or parchment paper.
2. Combine marinade ingredients in a small bowl.
3. Mix potatoes with 3 tablespoons of the marinade.
4. Place potatoes on baking sheet in a single layer and roast for 15 minutes.
5. While potatoes are cooking, toss asparagus with 2 tablespoons of the marinade.
6. Remove potatoes from oven, mix in asparagus and place salmon filets on top of vegetables.
7. Brush salmon with remaining marinade and return baking sheet to oven for about 10 minutes, or until salmon is firm.
8. Finish salmon under broiler to brown the fish, about 5 minutes.

Nutrition Facts

Balsamic-Glazed Salmon and Asparagus

Amount Per Serving

Calories 435	Calories from Fat 162

	% Daily Value*
Total Fat 18g	28%
Saturated Fat 3g	15%
Polyunsaturated Fat 5g	
Monounsaturated Fat 9g	
Cholesterol 94mg	31%
Sodium 280mg	12%
Potassium 1595mg	46%
Total Carbohydrates 29g	10%
Dietary Fiber 5g	20%
Sugars 9g	
Protein 39g	78%
Vitamin A	20%
Vitamin C	48%
Calcium	6%
Iron	27%

* Percent Daily Values are based on a 2000 calorie diet.

Cod, Tomatoes & Dill

Makes 4 servings

Make-Ahead Tip

The marinade can be made ahead of time, but fish is delicate enough that it is best cooked fresh and eaten immediately.

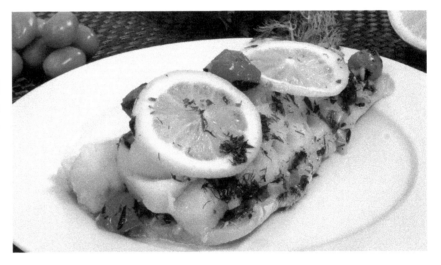

Ingredients

4 6-ounce cod filets
2 tablespoons olive oil
¼ teaspoon kosher salt
¼ teaspoon black pepper
½ cup celery, thinly sliced
½ cup cherry tomatoes, halved
½ cup fresh Italian parsley leaves, chopped and loosely packed
¼ cup fresh dill sprigs, chopped and loosely packed, divided
1 lemon, cut into 8 thin slices

Directions

1. Preheat oven to 400 degrees. Line a sheet pan with foil or parchment paper.
2. In a bowl, make the marinade by mixing olive oil, salt, pepper celery, tomatoes, parsley and 2 tablespoons of the chopped dill.
3. Cut a piece of parchment paper 28 inches long and place on the sheet pan.
4. Place half of the fish in the middle of the parchment paper; top fish with half of marinade mixture and 4 slices of the lemon.
5. Layer on remaining fish and top with remainder of marinade and lemon slices.
6. Fold in sides of parchment paper; bring long ends of paper together and fold 3 times to make a seam. Secure with a metal paper clip.
7. Bake until fish is opaque, about 12-15 minutes.
8. To serve, remove from parchment and top with remaining dill.

Nutrition Facts

Cod, Tomatoes and Dill

Amount Per Serving

Calories 213	Calories from Fat 72

	% Daily Value*
Total Fat 8g	12%
Saturated Fat 1g	5%
Polyunsaturated Fat 1g	
Monounsaturated Fat 5g	
Cholesterol 75mg	25%
Sodium 226mg	9%
Potassium 110mg	3%
Total Carbohydrates 4g	1%
Dietary Fiber 1g	4%
Sugars 1g	
Protein 31g	62%
Vitamin A	7%
Vitamin C	26%
Calcium	3%
Iron	5%

* Percent Daily Values are based on a 2000 calorie diet.

Turmeric-Basil Tilapia Bake

Makes 4 servings

Make-Ahead Tip
Cooked fish only keeps for a day or two in the refrigerator. Its texture deteriorates if frozen.

Prep Step
Since most fish cooks very quickly, it is best to prep your other ingredients in advance and cook the fish just before serving.

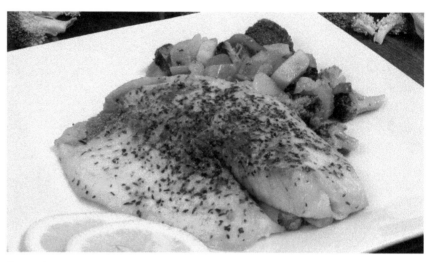

Nutrition Facts
Turmeric-Basil Tilapia Bake

Amount Per Serving

Calories 303	Calories from Fat 144

	% Daily Value*
Total Fat 16g	25%
Saturated Fat 3g	15%
Polyunsaturated Fat 1g	
Monounsaturated Fat 10g	
Cholesterol 75mg	25%
Sodium 381mg	16%
Potassium 17mg	0%
Total Carbohydrates 6g	2%
Dietary Fiber 2g	8%
Sugars 2g	
Protein 33g	66%
Vitamin A	2%
Vitamin C	34%
Calcium	3%
Iron	6%

* Percent Daily Values are based on a 2000 calorie diet.

Ingredients

24 ounces tilapia fillets
2 16-ounce bags frozen vegetable blend
 (broccoli, yellow squash, green beans, onions and red peppers)
¼ cup olive oil
1½ teaspoons dried basil
1½ teaspoons dried thyme
¾ teaspoon ground turmeric
¼ teaspoon garlic powder
¼ teaspoon black pepper
¼ teaspoon kosher salt

Directions

1. Preheat oven to 350 degrees. Line a sheet pan with foil or parchment paper.
2. Mix spices, except kosher salt, into olive oil.
3. Place tilapia and vegetables on sheet pan and baste well with olive oil mixture.
4. Bake 20-25 minutes, until fish reaches an internal temperature of 145 degrees.
5. Season to taste with kosher salt.
6. Serve over brown rice, quinoa or other whole grain, as desired.

Pork Stir-Fry

Makes 8 servings

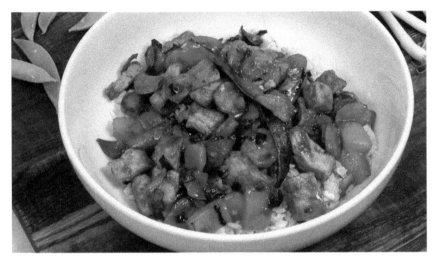

Ingredients

6 tablespoons sesame oil
3 pounds pork loin, sliced in thin pieces
2 tablespoons fresh ginger, minced
1 tablespoon garlic, minced
3 cups carrots, peeled and thinly sliced on the bias
3 cups red bell pepper, cut into strips
2 cups snow pea pods, ends trimmed
⅔ cup low-sodium teriyaki sauce
2 tablespoons water
2 tablespoons corn starch
½ cup green onion, thinly sliced
Crushed red pepper, optional
4 cups cooked brown rice, optional

Directions

1. Whisk together teriyaki sauce, cornstarch and water.
2. Heat oil in large skillet over medium-high heat.
3. Sauté pork loin, ginger, garlic and carrots until pork starts to brown, about 5-7 minutes. Work in batches if pan is too full.
4. Add red pepper and pea pods and continue cooking, stirring occasionally.
5. Once veggies are tender, stir in teriyaki mixture, add green onions and cook until sauce is reduced to desired thickness.
6. Sprinkle with crushed red pepper and serve with brown rice, as desired.

Nutrition Facts

Pork Stir Fry

Amount Per Serving

Calories 368	Calories from Fat 144

	% Daily Value*
Total Fat 16g	25%
Saturated Fat 4g	20%
Polyunsaturated Fat 5g	
Monounsaturated Fat 7g	
Cholesterol 111mg	37%
Sodium 512mg	21%
Potassium 1002mg	29%
Total Carbohydrates 16g	5%
Dietary Fiber 3g	12%
Sugars 8g	
Protein 39g	78%
Vitamin A	202%
Vitamin C	203%
Calcium	4%
Iron	19%

* Percent Daily Values are based on a 2000 calorie diet.

Pork Tenderloin and Brussels Sprouts

Makes 4 servings

Make-Ahead Tip
Keeps well in refrigerator for 2-3 days. Can be frozen, but the flavor and texture will not be quite as good as when it is fresh.

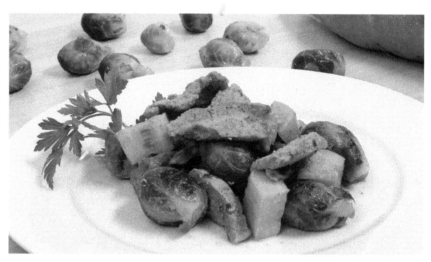

Ingredients

24 ounces pork tenderloin, thinly sliced

1 12-ounce bag frozen Brussels sprouts

3 cups sweet potatoes, diced

¼ cup unsalted butter, melted

1½ teaspoons chili powder

1½ teaspoons ground cumin

½ teaspoon garlic powder

½ teaspoon paprika

¼ teaspoon onion powder

¼ teaspoon kosher salt

Directions

1. Preheat oven to 375 degrees. Line a sheet pan with foil or parchment paper.
2. Mix spices into melted butter.
3. Place pork and vegetables on sheet pan. Baste well with butter mixture.
4. Bake 30 minutes or until pork reaches an internal temperature of 145 degrees. Allow to rest for at least 3 minutes after removing from oven.
5. Serve over brown rice, quinoa or other whole grain, as desired.

Nutrition Facts
Pork Tenderloin and Brussels Sprouts

Amount Per Serving

Calories 466	Calories from Fat 189

	% Daily Value*
Total Fat 21g	32%
Saturated Fat 11g	55%
Polyunsaturated Fat 2g	
Monounsaturated Fat 7g	
Cholesterol 145mg	48%
Sodium 231mg	10%
Potassium 1311mg	37%
Total Carbohydrates 28g	9%
Dietary Fiber 7g	28%
Sugars 4g	
Protein 40g	80%
Vitamin A	311%
Vitamin C	110%
Calcium	8%
Iron	22%

* Percent Daily Values are based on a 2000 calorie diet.

Slow Cooker & Multicooker Meals

Slow cookers are great: Add your ingredients in the morning, turn on the slow cooker and your meal is ready when you get home.

Instant Pots® and other multicookers are also used to make batch meals and can be used for slow cooking, but they also have a pressure cooker function that greatly shortens cooking times. Both are convenient ways to make quality meals easily.

Our recipes usually make larger quantities than can be used in one meal, so you will have food for several meals.

Hearty Slow Cooker Chicken Soup

Makes 6-8 servings

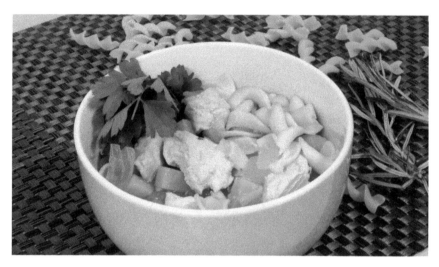

Ingredients

1 ½ pounds chicken breast, diced
2 cups carrots, diced
2 cups onion, diced
2 cups celery, chopped
3 tablespoons garlic, minced
3 tablespoons olive oil
½ teaspoon dried thyme
1 bay leaf
2 sprigs fresh rosemary
4 cups low-sodium chicken broth
½ teaspoon salt
2 cups water
2 cups dry whole wheat egg noodles*

Directions

1. Add all ingredients except pasta to slow cooker and mix together.
2. Cover and cook on low for 6-8 hours.
3. Discard bay leaf and rosemary sprigs.
4. Add pasta and cook for 20-30 minutes.

*Substitute enriched white flour egg noodles if whole wheat egg noodles are not available.

Nutrition Facts
Hearty Slow Cooker Chicken Soup

Amount Per Serving

Calories 230	Calories from Fat 63

	% Daily Value*
Total Fat 7g	11%
Saturated Fat 1g	5%
Polyunsaturated Fat 1g	
Monounsaturated Fat 4g	
Cholesterol 63mg	21%
Sodium 340mg	14%
Potassium 411mg	12%
Total Carbohydrates 19g	6%
Dietary Fiber 3g	12%
Sugars 5g	
Protein 24g	48%
Vitamin A	95%
Vitamin C	12%
Calcium	4%
Iron	3%

* Percent Daily Values are based on a 2000 calorie diet.

Slow Cooker Chicken Chili

Makes 6 servings

Recommended Toppings
Diced avocado
Finely seeded and diced
*   jalapeño pepper*
Chopped cilantro
Shredded cheese of choice
Greek yogurt
Tortilla chips

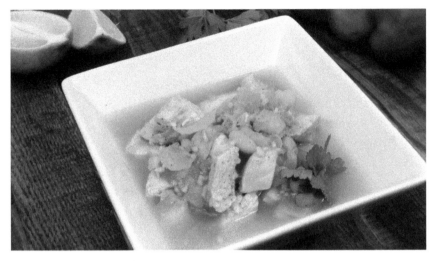

Nutrition Facts
Slow Cooker Chicken Chili

Amount Per Serving

Calories 351	Calories from Fat 9

	% Daily Value*
Total Fat 1g	2%
Saturated Fat 0.1g	1%
Polyunsaturated Fat 0.2g	
Monounsaturated Fat 0.2g	
Cholesterol 65mg	22%
Sodium 506mg	21%
Potassium 348mg	10%
Total Carbohydrates 44g	15%
Dietary Fiber 15g	60%
Sugars 1g	
Protein 40g	80%
Vitamin A	7%
Vitamin C	19%
Calcium	11%
Iron	30%

* Percent Daily Values are based on a 2000 calorie diet.

Ingredients
1½ pounds chicken breast, diced
4 cups low-sodium chicken broth
4 14.5-ounce cans Great Northern white beans, rinsed, drained
1 cup onion, chopped
¼ cup garlic, minced
1 4.5-ounce can diced green chilis
2 tablespoons lime juice
1 tablespoon cumin
2 teaspoons chili powder
¼ teaspoon cayenne pepper
½ teaspoon salt
¼ teaspoon black pepper

Directions
1. Mash half of the beans with a potato masher or blender.
2. Place diced chicken breast in bottom of slow cooker, add remaining ingredients and mix ingredients together.
3. Cover and cook on low for 5-6 hours until chicken is cooked.
4. Serve with your choice of toppings and tortilla chips.

Slow Cooker Cheesy Lentils

Makes 10-15 servings

Make-Ahead Tip
Portion into single-serving containers and refrigerate for several days or freeze for several months for grab-and-go convenience.

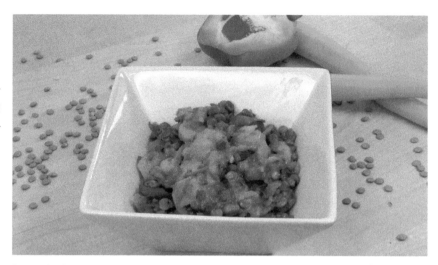

Ingredients
4 cups low-sodium vegetable or chicken broth
1 pound dry green or yellow lentils, rinsed
1 large yellow onion, chopped small
3 large carrots, thinly sliced
1 tablespoon garlic, minced
1 teaspoon salt
¼ teaspoon black pepper
½ teaspoon dried leaf thyme
1 14.5-ounce can diced tomatoes, drained
1 4-ounce can diced green chilis, drained
1½ cups bell pepper (any color), chopped
¾ teaspoon dried leaf parsley
1 8-ounce package extra sharp shredded cheddar cheese
1 pound chicken breast, cooked and chopped (optional)

Directions for Making in a Slow Cooker
1. Combine all ingredients except shredded cheese in slow cooker. Cover and cook on low for 5-6 hours or until lentils are tender.
2. Sprinkle cheese on top; cover slow cooker to melt cheese.

Directions for Making in the Oven
1. Preheat oven to 350 degrees.
2. In a 13x9x2-inch baking dish, combine all ingredients except the cheese. Cover with foil and bake for 90 minutes or until lentils are tender. This can be made in advance.
3. Stir thoroughly and sprinkle cheese on top. Bake, uncovered, for 5-10 minutes or until cheese is melted.

Nutrition Facts
Slow Cooker Cheesy Lentils

Amount Per Serving

Calories 311	Calories from Fat 72

	% Daily Value*
Total Fat 8g	12%
Saturated Fat 4g	20%
Polyunsaturated Fat 0.1g	
Monounsaturated Fat 0.02g	
Cholesterol 24mg	8%
Sodium 353mg	15%
Potassium 757mg	22%
Total Carbohydrates 40g	13%
Dietary Fiber 17g	68%
Sugars 6g	
Protein 20g	40%
Vitamin A	117%
Vitamin C	142%
Calcium	21%
Iron	23%

* Percent Daily Values are based on a 2000 calorie diet.

Slow Cooker Mexican Quinoa

Makes 8 servings

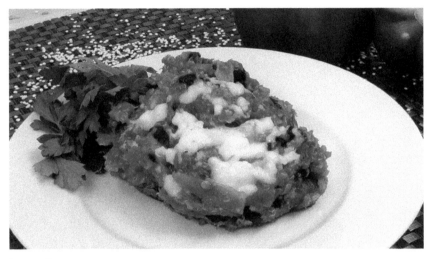

Ingredients

1 cup onion, chopped
1 ½ cups dry quinoa
2 cups Southwestern Sauce (recipe on page 71) or taco sauce
2 15-ounce cans low-sodium black beans, rinsed and drained
1 15-ounce can diced tomatoes
1 large red bell pepper, diced
1 large green bell pepper, diced
½ teaspoon salt
¾ cup water
1 cup shredded Mexican cheese blend or queso fresco or cojita

Directions

1. Place all ingredients (except cheese) in slow cooker. Stir to combine.
2. Cover and cook on low for 4-5 hours until liquid is absorbed and quinoa is tender.
3. Stir in half of the shredded cheese, and sprinkle remaining cheese over top.
4. Cover and cook on high for 15 minutes, until cheese melts.

Nutrition Facts

Slow Cooker Mexican Quinoa

Amount Per Serving

Calories 307	Calories from Fat 54

	% Daily Value*
Total Fat 6g	**9%**
Saturated Fat 2g	**10%**
Polyunsaturated Fat 0.3g	
Monounsaturated Fat 0.2g	
Cholesterol 9mg	**3%**
Sodium 271mg	**11%**
Potassium 547mg	**16%**
Total Carbohydrates 51g	**17%**
Dietary Fiber 12g	**48%**
Sugars 8g	
Protein 15g	**30%**
Vitamin A	38%
Vitamin C	150%
Calcium	14%
Iron	26%

* Percent Daily Values are based on a 2000 calorie diet.

Slow Cooker Breakfast Casserole

Makes 8 servings

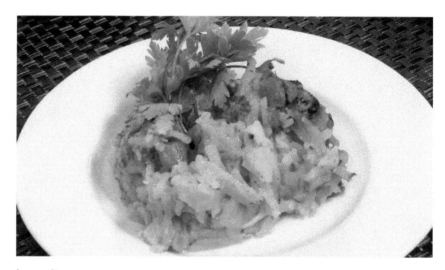

Ingredients

1 ½ pounds cooked chicken breast, diced (leftover is fine)

1 20-ounce package shredded hash brown potatoes
(sold in refrigerated section; if using frozen, thaw and squeeze
out excess moisture with paper towels)

1 teaspoon garlic powder or granulated garlic

½ teaspoon thyme

1 teaspoon paprika

1 pound frozen broccoli

2 cups shredded sharp cheddar cheese, divided

½ teaspoon salt

Directions

1. Mix together chicken, hash browns, garlic, thyme, paprika,
   broccoli and 1 ½ cups cheese.
2. Oil the bottom of the slow cooker, add the chicken and potato
   mixture and top with the remaining cheese.
3. Cook on high for 1 hour; reduce heat to low and cook for 4
   additional hours.

Nutrition Facts

Slow Cooker Breakfast Casserole

Amount Per Serving

Calories 240	Calories from Fat 72

	% Daily Value*
Total Fat 8g	12%
Saturated Fat 4g	20%
Polyunsaturated Fat 0.02g	
Monounsaturated Fat 2g	
Cholesterol 68mg	23%
Sodium 340mg	14%
Potassium 459mg	13%
Total Carbohydrates 15g	5%
Dietary Fiber 2g	8%
Sugars 1g	
Protein 27g	54%
Vitamin A	7%
Vitamin C	13%
Calcium	16%
Iron	6%

* Percent Daily Values are based on a 2000 calorie
diet.

Slow Cooker Mozzarella Eggplant

Makes 6 servings

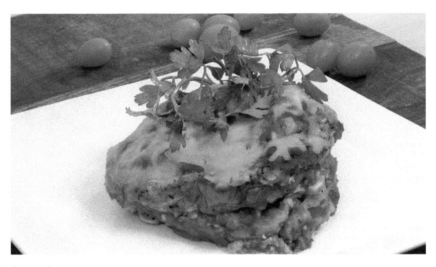

Ingredients

1½ cups bread crumbs
1½ teaspoons dried basil, divided
1½ teaspoons dried oregano, divided
1½ teaspoons dried thyme, divided
2½ teaspoons garlic powder, divided
¾ teaspoon salt
½ teaspoon black pepper
1 29-ounce can tomato purée
2 large- or 3 medium-sized eggplants, peeled, cut in ½-inch slices
3 eggs, lightly whisked
2 cups mozzarella cheese, shredded

Directions

1. Mix bread crumbs with ½ teaspoon each of the basil, oregano, thyme, and garlic powder.
2. Combine remaining basil, oregano, thyme, garlic powder, salt and pepper with tomato purée in a separate bowl.
3. Spread ¼ cup sauce on bottom of slow cooker.
4. Dip eggplant pieces in egg wash, then coat with bread crumbs. Place a layer of dipped eggplant pieces over the sauce.
5. Cover eggplant layer with ¼ cup sauce and then sprinkle with ½ cup cheese.
6. Repeat process until all ingredients are layered, ending with cheese on top. In a large slow cooker, this is 2-3 layers.
7. Place lid on slow cooker and cook on low for 5-6 hours, until eggplant is tender and cheese is melted.

Nutrition Facts

Slow Cooker Mozzarella Eggplant

Amount Per Serving

Calories 252	Calories from Fat 90

	% Daily Value*
Total Fat 10g	15%
Saturated Fat 5g	25%
Polyunsaturated Fat 14g	
Monounsaturated Fat 3g	
Cholesterol 126mg	42%
Sodium 502mg	21%
Potassium 97mg	3%
Total Carbohydrates 34g	11%
Dietary Fiber 10g	40%
Sugars 8g	
Protein 19g	38%
Vitamin A	28%
Vitamin C	37%
Calcium	32%
Iron	16%

* Percent Daily Values are based on a 2000 calorie diet.

Slow Cooker Shredded Pork

Makes 8 servings

Cooking Tip

If using a multicooker, brown the meat in the multicooker on the sauté setting and then continue as directed.

Recommended Toppings

Diced tomatoes
Chopped cilantro
Sliced radishes
Shredded cheese of choice
Lime wedges

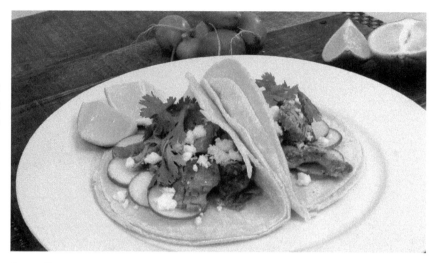

Nutrition Facts

Slow Cooker Shredded Pork

Amount Per Serving

Calories 625	Calories from Fat 405

	% Daily Value*
Total Fat 45g	69%
Saturated Fat 80g	400%
Polyunsaturated Fat 5g	
Monounsaturated Fat 20g	
Cholesterol 160mg	53%
Sodium 501mg	21%
Potassium 785mg	22%
Total Carbohydrates 15g	5%
Dietary Fiber 8g	32%
Sugars 1g	
Protein 45g	90%
Vitamin A	7%
Vitamin C	15%
Calcium	9%
Iron	27%

* Percent Daily Values are based on a 2000 calorie diet.

Ingredients

1 tablespoon olive oil
2 tablespoons lime juice (approx. 1 lime)
2 tablespoons garlic, minced
1 tablespoon chili powder
1 tablespoon cumin
1 tablespoon dried oregano
1 teaspoon dried thyme
½ teaspoon salt
½ teaspoon black pepper
1 pork shoulder (4-5 pounds), trimmed of excess fat
1 cup low-sodium chicken broth
1 cup onion, chopped
1 4.5-ounce can green chilis
1 bay leaf
8 whole wheat or 16 corn tortillas (2 corn tortillas per taco)

Directions

1. Mix together olive oil, lime juice, garlic, spices (except bay leaf), and salt and pepper and rub on pork shoulder.
2. In large pan, heat oil over high heat and sear pork on each side.
3. Place pork in slow cooker and add broth, onions, green chilis and bay leaf. Cook on low for 8 hours, or until pork is tender.
4. Remove pork from slow cooker and shred. Remove bay leaf and return pork to slow cooker on warm setting for serving.
5. Portion shredded pork and desired toppings on tortillas.

Slow Cooker Turkey Spinach Lasagna

Makes 8 servings

Make-Ahead Tip
Freeze extra meat sauce. Defrost to speed dinner preparation on busy evenings.

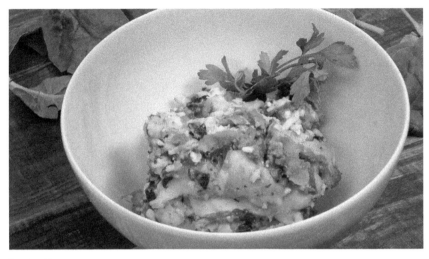

Nutrition Facts

Slow Cooker Lasagna

Amount Per Serving

Calories 548	Calories from Fat 189

	% Daily Value*
Total Fat 21g	32%
Saturated Fat 10g	50%
Polyunsaturated Fat 1g	
Monounsaturated Fat 4g	
Cholesterol 80mg	27%
Sodium 318mg	13%
Potassium 257mg	7%
Total Carbohydrates 48g	16%
Dietary Fiber 8g	32%
Sugars 15g	
Protein 49g	98%
Vitamin A	155%
Vitamin C	47%
Calcium	55%
Iron	128%

* Percent Daily Values are based on a 2000 calorie diet.

Ingredients
2 tablespoons olive oil
2 pounds ground turkey
2 cups onion, diced
1 12-ounce package frozen spinach, thawed
2 29-ounce cans low-sodium tomato purée
1½ teaspoons dried basil
1½ teaspoons dried oregano
1½ teaspoons garlic powder
1½ teaspoons dried thyme
¾ teaspoon salt
2½ cups ricotta or cottage cheese
8 ounces shredded mozzarella cheese
12 uncooked whole wheat or gluten-free lasagna noodles,
   broken in half

Directions
1. Heat oil in a large skillet on medium-high heat. Cook ground turkey and onions until turkey is cooked through and no longer pink, about 5 minutes.
2. Add spices, salt and tomato purée and cook for 5 minutes.
3. Combine cheeses and spinach together in a mixing bowl.
4. Spread ⅓ of the meat sauce on bottom of slow cooker.
5. Cover sauce with ⅓ of the lasagna noodles.
6. Spread ⅓ of the cheese mixture over noodles. Repeat until all ingredients are used, ending with a layer of cheese.
7. Cover and cook on low heat until noodles are al dente, 5-6 hours.

Hearty Multicooker Pot Roast

Makes 8 servings

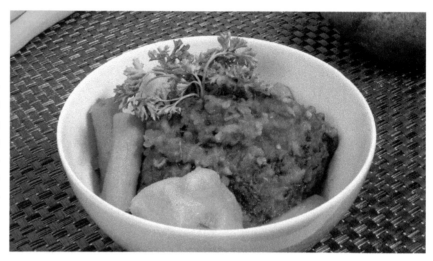

Make-Ahead Tip
The perfect dish for batch cooking! Store cooked meal with the vegetables on the bottom on the storage container in the pan juices and they will absorb even more flavor. Reheat for a quick and tasty weeknight meal that melts in your mouth!

Serving Tip
Remove roast and vegetables from pot and serve on a deep platter with the cooking juices.

Nutrition Facts
Hearty Multicooker Pot Roast

Amount Per Serving

Calories 645	Calories from Fat 315

	% Daily Value*
Total Fat 35g	54%
Saturated Fat 13g	65%
Polyunsaturated Fat 2g	
Monounsaturated Fat 16g	
Cholesterol 116mg	39%
Sodium 400mg	17%
Potassium 1601mg	46%
Total Carbohydrates 43g	14%
Dietary Fiber 7g	28%
Sugars 7g	
Protein 38g	76%
Vitamin A	382%
Vitamin C	69%
Calcium	8%
Iron	26%

* Percent Daily Values are based on a 2000 calorie diet.

Ingredients
3 pounds beef chuck roast, trimmed of excess fat
1 teaspoon salt, divided
½ teaspoon black pepper, divided
2 tablespoon olive oil
2 cups low-sodium beef broth
2 tablespoons minced garlic
2 tablespoons Worcestershire sauce
¼ teaspoon Tabasco sauce
1 teaspoon dried oregano
1 teaspoon dried thyme
3 pounds yellow potatoes, cut in 2-inch chunks
2 pounds carrots, peeled and cut in 3-inch lengths
2 pounds yellow onion, quartered

Directions
1. Season roast with ¼ teaspoon salt and ⅛ teaspoon pepper.
2. Heat multicooker on sauté setting, add oil and brown meat well on both sides—about 5-7 minutes per side. Remove from pot.
3. Deglaze the pan by adding the broth, garlic, spices and herbs. Place 4 onion pieces on bottom of pot and place meat on top of them. Fasten lid, turn steam valve to sealed setting and set multicooker to pressure cook (manual setting) for 50 minutes.
4. When cycle is complete, manually release the pressure and remove the lid. Layer the vegetables on top of the meat in this order: potatoes, carrots, onions. Season each layer with salt and pepper. Replace lid, ensure steam valve is sealed, and set the multicooker to pressure cook for 20 minutes.
5. When the second cycle ends, release pressure manually.

Slow Cooker Beef & Barley Stew

Makes 6 servings

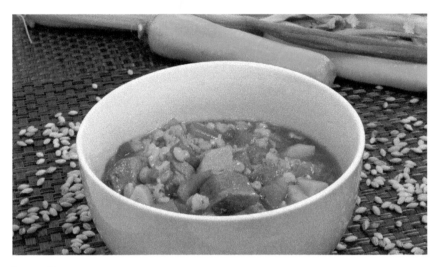

Ingredients

1 tablespoon olive oil
2 pounds chuck roast, trimmed of excess fat, cubed
1 ½ cups carrots, peeled and diced
1 ½ cups celery, diced
1 cup onion
¾ cup pearled barley
2 bay leaves
½ teaspoon dried thyme
½ teaspoon salt
¾ teaspoon black pepper
2 teaspoons fresh lemon juice, or to taste
6 cups low-sodium beef broth

Directions

1. Preheat slow cooker on high setting.
2. In large skillet, heat oil on medium-high heat and brown the beef. Add the browned beef to slow cooker.
3. Pour 1 cup of broth into skillet and deglaze pan; add liquid to slow cooker.
4. Add carrots, celery, onions, barley, remaining broth and spices and stir.
5. Turn heat to low, cover and cook for 6 hours.
6. Just before serving, stir in the fresh lemon juice.

Nutrition Facts

Slow Cooker Beef and Barley Stew

Amount Per Serving

Calories 352	Calories from Fat 81
	% Daily Value*
Total Fat 9g	**14%**
Saturated Fat 3g	**15%**
Polyunsaturated Fat 1g	
Monounsaturated Fat 4g	
Cholesterol 67mg	**22%**
Sodium 391mg	**16%**
Potassium 790mg	**23%**
Total Carbohydrates 27g	**9%**
Dietary Fiber 6g	**24%**
Sugars 4g	
Protein 40g	**80%**
Vitamin A	110%
Vitamin C	8%
Calcium	8%
Iron	24%

* Percent Daily Values are based on a 2000 calorie diet.

Dressings & Sauces

Store-bought dressings and sauces are usually full of bad fats, added sugar, chemicals and artificial colors—this is why many of them can be kept for as long as a year without spoiling! They are some of the most highly processed foods in your kitchen.

While homemade sauces and dressings last only about a week before spoiling, they can be quickly and easily made in small batches and are tastier and far healthier for you than most commercial brands. You will be surprised by how much they improve the taste of your food and ask yourself why you didn't start making them from scratch years ago!

Asian Vinaigrette

Makes 1½ cups or 12 2-Tbsp servings

Nutrition Facts

Asian Vinaigrette

Amount Per Serving

Calories 166	Calories from Fat 162
	% Daily Value*
Total Fat 18g	**28%**
Saturated Fat 2g	**10%**
Polyunsaturated Fat 2g	
Monounsaturated Fat 13g	
Sodium 101mg	**4%**
Potassium 8mg	**0%**
Total Carbohydrates 2g	**1%**
Dietary Fiber 0.04g	**0%**
Sugars 1g	
Protein 0.2g	**0%**
Vitamin C	0.1%
Calcium	0.1%
Iron	1%

* Percent Daily Values are based on a 2000 calorie diet.

Ingredients

¼ cup apple cider vinegar

2 tablespoons low-sodium soy sauce or tamari sauce

1 cup extra-virgin olive oil

2 tablespoons honey

½ teaspoon ground ginger

¼ teaspoon black pepper, or to taste

Directions

1. Combine all ingredients in a bowl and whisk vigorously. Or, place all ingredients in a leak-proof jar and shake vigorously.

Citrus Vinaigrette

Makes 1 cup or 8 2-Tbsp servings

Nutrition Facts

Citrus Vinaigrette

Amount Per Serving

Calories 160	Calories from Fat 162
	% Daily Value*
Total Fat 18g	**28%**
Saturated Fat 2g	**10%**
Polyunsaturated Fat 2g	
Monounsaturated Fat 13g	
Sodium 20mg	**1%**
Potassium 13mg	**0%**
Total Carbohydrates 1g	**0%**
Dietary Fiber 0.1g	**0%**
Sugars 0.2g	
Protein 0.1g	**0%**
Vitamin A	0.2%
Vitamin C	4%
Calcium	0.1%
Iron	1%

* Percent Daily Values are based on a 2000 calorie diet.

Ingredients

⅓ cup lemon or lime juice (2 lemons or 3 limes)

⅔ cup extra virgin olive oil

1½ teaspoons dried parsley

⅛ teaspoon salt, or to taste

⅛ teaspoon black pepper, or to taste

Directions

1. Combine all ingredients in a bowl and whisk vigorously. Or, place all ingredients in a leak-proof jar and shake vigorously.

Dijon Vinaigrette

Makes 1 cup or 8 2-Tbsp servings

Nutrition Facts

Dijon Vingaigrette

Amount Per Serving

Calories 126	Calories from Fat 126

	% Daily Value*
Total Fat 14g	**22%**
Saturated Fat 2g	**10%**
Polyunsaturated Fat 1g	
Monounsaturated Fat 10g	
Sodium 126mg	**5%**
Potassium 23mg	**1%**
Total Carbohydrates 1g	**0%**
Dietary Fiber 0.3g	**1%**
Sugars 0.4g	
Protein 0.3g	**1%**
Vitamin C	5%
Calcium	0.4%
Iron	1%

* Percent Daily Values are based on a 2000 calorie diet.

Ingredients

2 tablespoons Dijon mustard
2 teaspoons garlic, minced
6 tablespoons lemon juice
½ cup extra virgin olive oil
¼ teaspoon salt, or to taste
¼ teaspoon black pepper, or to taste

Directions

1. Combine mustard, garlic, vinegar and lemon juice in a bowl.
2. Drizzle in the oil while whisking continuously and season with salt and pepper.
3. Or, place all ingredients in a leak-proof jar and shake vigorously until combined.

Raspberry Vinaigrette

Makes 1 cup or 8 2-Tbsp servings

Nutrition Facts

Raspberry Balsamic Vinaigrette

Amount Per Serving

Calories 183	Calories from Fat 180

	% Daily Value*
Total Fat 20g	**31%**
Saturated Fat 3g	**15%**
Polyunsaturated Fat 2g	
Monounsaturated Fat 14g	
Sodium 60mg	**3%**
Potassium 25mg	**1%**
Total Carbohydrates 2g	**1%**
Dietary Fiber 1g	**4%**
Sugars 1g	
Protein 0.2g	**0%**
Vitamin A	0.1%
Vitamin C	7%
Calcium	0.4%
Iron	1%

* Percent Daily Values are based on a 2000 calorie diet.

Ingredients

½ cup raspberries, fresh or frozen
¼ tablespoon balsamic vinegar
¼ teaspoon salt
¼ teaspoon pepper
⅔ cup extra virgin olive oil

Directions

1. Place all ingredients except olive oil in a blender and pulse until thoroughly combined.
2. With blender running slowly, add olive oil and blend until emulsified.
3. To make by hand, crush berries in a bowl. Transfer berries and remaining ingredients to a container with a leak-proof lid and shake vigorously until well blended.

Turmeric Vinaigrette

Makes 1 cup or 8 2-Tbsp servings

Nutrition Facts
Turmeric Vinaigrette

Amount Per Serving

Calories 129	Calories from Fat 126
	% Daily Value*
Total Fat 14g	**22%**
Saturated Fat 2g	**10%**
Polyunsaturated Fat 1g	
Monounsaturated Fat 10g	
Sodium 37mg	**2%**
Potassium 46mg	**1%**
Total Carbohydrates 2g	**1%**
Dietary Fiber 0.2g	**1%**
Sugars 2g	
Protein 0.2g	**0%**
Vitamin A	1%
Vitamin C	13%
Calcium	0.2%
Iron	2%

* Percent Daily Values are based on a 2000 calorie diet.

Ingredients

2 teaspoon ground turmeric
½ cup fresh-squeezed orange juice
2 teaspoons balsamic vinegar
2 teaspoons honey, optional
⅛ teaspoon salt, or to taste
⅛ teaspoon pepper, or to taste
½ cup extra virgin olive oil

Directions

1. Place all ingredients except olive oil in a bowl and mix well.
2. Add olive oil and whisk vigorously until mixture is well blended.
3. Alternate method: Place all ingredients in a leak-proof jar and shake vigorously.
4. Allow flavor to develop for at least 30 minutes before serving.

Avocado Dressing

Makes 1 cup or 8 2-Tbsp servings

Nutrition Facts
Avocado Dressing

Amount Per Serving

Calories 55	Calories from Fat 45
	% Daily Value*
Total Fat 5g	**8%**
Saturated Fat 1g	**5%**
Polyunsaturated Fat 1g	
Monounsaturated Fat 4g	
Cholesterol 0.3mg	**0%**
Sodium 156mg	**7%**
Potassium 125mg	**4%**
Total Carbohydrates 2g	**1%**
Dietary Fiber 1g	**4%**
Sugars 1g	
Protein 1g	**2%**
Vitamin A	18%
Vitamin C	10%
Calcium	2%
Iron	2%

* Percent Daily Values are based on a 2000 calorie diet.

Ingredients

½ ripe avocado
2 tablespoons extra virgin olive oil
¼ cup plain Greek yogurt, regular or low-fat
½ cup water
1 small bunch cilantro leaves and stems, minced
1 tablespoon fresh lime juice (½ lime)
1 jalapeño pepper, seeded
½ teaspoon salt, or to taste

Directions

1. Combine all ingredients in a blender and pulse until smooth.
2. To make by hand, mash avocado, add remaining ingredients and whisk vigorously.
3. If dressing is too thick, add more water. If dressing is too thin, add more avocado.

Lemon Cumin Yogurt Sauce

Makes 1 cup or 8 2-Tbsp servings

Nutrition Facts
Lemon Cumin Yogurt Sauce

Amount Per Serving

Calories 16

	% Daily Value*
Total Fat 0.01g	0%
Saturated Fat 0.002g	0%
Polyunsaturated Fat 0.002g	
Monounsaturated Fat 0.01g	
Cholesterol 1mg	0%
Sodium 15mg	1%
Potassium 10mg	0%
Total Carbohydrates 1g	0%
Dietary Fiber 0.1g	0%
Sugars 1g	
Protein 3g	6%
Vitamin A	3%
Vitamin C	5%
Calcium	4%
Iron	3%

* Percent Daily Values are based on a 2000 calorie diet.

Ingredients

1 cup plain Greek yogurt, regular or low-fat
4 teaspoons fresh lemon juice
2 teaspoons ground cumin
¼ cup Italian parsley, minced

Directions

1. Place all ingredients in a bowl and mix well.
2. Allow flavor to develop for at least 30 minutes before serving.

Lemon Dill Sauce

Makes 1 cup or 8 2-Tbsp servings

Nutrition Facts
Lemon Dill Sauce

Amount Per Serving

Calories 29	Calories from Fat 18
	% Daily Value*
Total Fat 2g	3%
Saturated Fat 1g	5%
Polyunsaturated Fat 0.003g	
Monounsaturated Fat 0.03g	
Cholesterol 6mg	2%
Sodium 166mg	7%
Potassium 84mg	2%
Total Carbohydrates 2g	1%
Dietary Fiber 0.1g	0%
Sugars 2g	
Protein 1g	2%
Vitamin A	7%
Vitamin C	6%
Calcium	5%
Iron	1%

* Percent Daily Values are based on a 2000 calorie diet.

Ingredients

2 teaspoons lemon juice
1 cup plain Greek yogurt, regular or low-fat
2 tablespoons fresh dill, minced
½ teaspoon salt

Directions

1. Combine ingredients in a small bowl and mix well.
2. Allow flavor to develop for at least 30 minutes before serving.

Ranch Dressing

Makes 1 cup or 8 2-Tbsp servings

Nutrition Facts
Ranch Dressing

Amount Per Serving

Calories 125	Calories from Fat 117

	% Daily Value*
Total Fat 13g	20%
Saturated Fat 1g	5%
Polyunsaturated Fat 0.002g	
Monounsaturated Fat 0.001g	
Cholesterol 13mg	4%
Sodium 103mg	4%
Potassium 23mg	1%
Total Carbohydrates 1g	0%
Dietary Fiber 0.1g	0%
Sugars 1g	
Protein 1g	2%
Vitamin A	1%
Vitamin C	1%
Calcium	2%
Iron	0.2%

* Percent Daily Values are based on a 2000 calorie diet.

Ingredients
1 tablespoon lemon juice
½ cup full-fat or low-fat Greek yogurt (do not use non-fat)
½ cup mayonnaise (avoid brands made with soybean oil)
⅛ teaspoon kosher or sea salt
⅛ teaspoon black pepper
½ teaspoon onion powder
½ teaspoon garlic powder or granulated garlic
⅛ teaspoon dried basil

Directions
1. Combine all ingredients thoroughly.
2. Allow flavor to develop for at least 30 minutes before serving.

Southwestern Sauce

Makes 2 cups or 16 2-Tbsp servings

Nutrition Facts
Southwestern Sauce

Amount Per Serving

Calories 19	Calories from Fat 2

	% Daily Value*
Total Fat 0.2g	0%
Saturated Fat 0.03g	0%
Polyunsaturated Fat 0.1g	
Monounsaturated Fat 0.1g	
Sodium 14mg	1%
Potassium 160mg	5%
Total Carbohydrates 4g	1%
Dietary Fiber 1g	4%
Sugars 2g	
Protein 1g	2%
Vitamin A	7%
Vitamin C	6%
Calcium	1%
Iron	5%

* Percent Daily Values are based on a 2000 calorie diet.

Ingredients
2 cups tomato purée
1½ teaspoons honey
1 tablespoon cumin
1 tablespoon chili powder
2 teaspoons granulated garlic or garlic powder
1¼ teaspoons onion powder
½ teaspoon cayenne pepper

Directions
1. Place all ingredients in a saucepan and vigorously whisk to combine.
2. Bring to a simmer and cook for 30 minutes to blend flavors.
3. Cool, bottle and refrigerate.

Smart Nutrition Tools & Resources

Chef Marshall's Meal-Planning Website

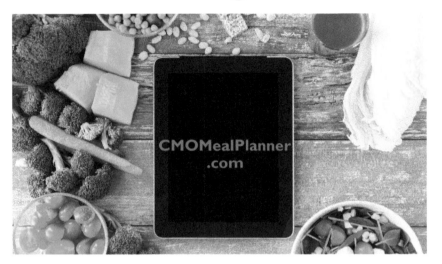

Our Smart Nutrition Meal-Planning Website—<u>SmartNutrition. Solutions</u>—makes it easy to save time while planning and preparing delicious, nutritious meals. Choose from dozens of recipes, plan your week's menu and print out your grocery list. Our site contains:

- **Delicious recipes** - New recipes added frequently.

- **Helpful planning tool** - We make it easy to plan your menus.

- **Instant shopping list** - With the touch of a button, you can print out a shopping list for single recipes, special event meals or for your entire week.

- **Health benefits** - Each recipe indicates its specific health benefits, such as reducing stress or improving the immune system.

- **Nutrition at a glance** - Each recipe includes a nutrition label plus nutrition totals for the day's menu.

To learn more or to sign up for the website, go to:

CMOMealPlanner.com

The Smart Nutrition Workbook

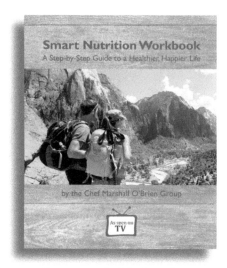

If you haven't yet discovered this handy resource, **The Smart Nutrition Workbook** is a companion guide to this cookbook and meal planner. It was written in response to our clients, who told us the biggest obstacle they faced in making changes that lead to a healthier lifestyle was in not knowing what to do or how to get started.

The Smart Nutrition Workbook provides a roadmap for those changes. It is a step-by-step guide to learning positive, energizing behaviors in the four most important areas of health—nutrition, sleep, hydration and physical activity.

Used in tandem with **The Smart Nutrition Cookbook & Meal Planner**, it will jump-start your journey to a healthier, happier you!

Learn more at:

www.SmartNutritionWorkbook.com

Smart Nutrition Meal Planning Template							
	Monday	Tuesday	Wednesday	Thursday	Friday	Saturday	Sunday
Breakfast							
Lunch							
Snack							
Dinner							

Conclusion

We know that people are short of time these days, so poor food choices are often made just to get people fed. It doesn't have to be this way. **The Smart Nutrition Cookbook & Meal Planner** is designed to give you cooking tips and recipes that help you start eating smart in the limited time you have. The recipes can be made quickly or prepared in advance for grab-and-go convenience. We tried to make everything simple, quick and delicious to nourish you and your family, not just feed you!

This only works if you do some planning. Each week you need to plan your meals and set aside some time on (or before) the weekend to shop so you can batch cook. Just imagine how great it will feel to come home and have a tasty and nutritious meal ready in minutes. Or, for those who think of batch cooking as "leftovers", prepare long-cooking ingredients—such as rice or beans—on the weekend and quickly do the final cooking on a weeknight for a freshly cooked meal.

We have also provided practical lists of the knives, pans, tools, food staples and spices with which you should stock your kitchen to make home cooking easy and quick. As you expand your skills, you can expand your list of tools and ingredients.

The Smart Nutrition Cookbook & Meal Planner gives you the tools to succeed. We hope you will enjoy the journey and know you will love the way the "new you" feels!

About the Authors

The Chef Marshall O'Brien Group's mission is to educate and empower people to achieve quality lives through smart nutrition. We strive to teach people that nourishing is different from eating. When we eat nourishing food, we perform better in everything we do.

The group is made up of chefs, dietitians, researchers, writers and videographers. The role of the researchers and dietitians is to understand current best nutrition practices and translate these practices into the right foods that produce the desired results. Since people will only eat the right foods if they taste good, our chefs use the recommended foods to create recipes that taste great. We call this "Putting Delicious in Nutritious."

The Chef Marshall O'Brien Group works with child care providers, schools, the YMCA, fire, police and public works departments, cities and corporations on staff wellness and nutrition strategies that help all people perform better.

In producing this book, we hope we have provided tools that will help everyone succeed in finding their pathway to a happier, healthier life.

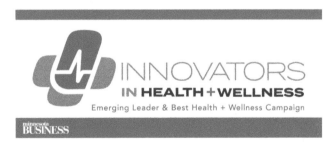